ChildBirth UNMASKED

ChildBirth UNMASKED

Margaret Jowitt

Published in 1993 by
Peter Wooller
Walford Lodge
Craven Arms
Shrops SY7 0JT

in conjunction with Peter Wooller

British Library Cataloguing in Publication Data

A catalogue record for this book is available from the British Library

PAPERBACK ISBN   0 9517691 3 8
HARDBACK ISBN   0 9517691 2 X

Printed and bound in Great Britain by Hartnolls Ltd, Bodmin, Cornwall.

Dedication

In memory of my mother and my mother-in-law

For all mothers, and for those who are with them in labour

Contents

Acknowledgments

This book owes its existence to Robin, my third-born and to Rosalind, the midwife who delivered him at less than a day's notice. Between them they allowed me to have the time of my life.

I owe my husband Robert a debt which I can never repay in giving me time to research, time to write, and encouragement when both tasks seemed impossible. He and the children have endured the conversion of a wife and mother into an author with great fortitude and must be pleased that it is all over now bar the shouting.

I would like to thank all those people who have taken the trouble to talk to me about their own knowledge of pregnancy and childbirth, be it practical or theoretical. While most of the research presented herein falls outside the confines of my official research, I would like to thank Professor S J Hutt and Dr P Chevins of the University of Keele for their interest and support. I would also like to thank the librarians at Keele, the North Staffs Medical Institute, and my local library for helping me to gain access to various books and articles.

I must thank Anne Voysey for reading an original draft and making helpful suggestions, for Christine Swain for much needed reassurance, and my husband and father for scrutinizing the final version before I committed myself to print. Special thanks are owed to Chris Redman at the SPA for interpreting some of my rough sketches and giving me the phrase "elastic memory" to describe my understanding of the directive forces of the uterus. Other illustrations represent the combined efforts of my husband, myself and the computer. I am very grateful for permission to reproduce the cartoons by Polly Ferguson on pages 163 and 187.

It would be quite impossible to list all who have influenced me, such a list would include most of the books I have read in my life, but three books in particular led to my theories about the role of stress hormones in pregnancy and labour: *Endogenous Substances Affecting the Myometrium*, the report of a symposium given under the auspices of The Endocrinological Society in 1965 about prostaglandins and how uterine muscle works; *Progesterone and the Defence Mechanism of Pregnancy*, a report of a symposium about Csapo's "Progesterone Block Hypothesis" given under the auspices of the CIBA Foundation in 1961, and *The Anatomy of a Scientific Discovery*, by Jeff Goldberg. The first I came across by chance in a secondhand bookshop at a stage when I had only just learned what the myometrium is, and the second I found in the Keele library, and the third I bought almost by chance when wanting light reading for the weekend. The rest of the work would have been impossible without the help of *Index Medicus*, a computerised listing of recent research findings in the medical sciences.

Apologia

I must apologise to those who feel that their own work has been used in an attempt to prove that 1 + 1 = 3, but must give them a gentle reminder that in respect of childbirth it does just that.

Short quotations have been taken from four books written by obstetricians, two of which were written for the lay readership. Derek Llewellyn-Jones' standard textbook happened to be the one I used in order to try to see childbirth from the medical viewpoint. My apologies to the authors concerned for using their particular words to highlight attitudes of their colleagues in general towards pregnancy, stress and labouring women.

Pregnancy, by Gordon Bourne, published by Pan in 1989.

The Fundamentals of Obstetrics and Gynaecology, part 1 Obstetrics, by Derek Llewellyn-Jones, published by Faber and Faber in 1990.

The Active Management of Labour, by Keiron O'Driscoll and Declan Meagher, published by Ballière Tindall in 1986.

Caesareans, by Elliott Philipps, published by Sidgwick and Jackson in 1988.

The author strongly recommends that mothers-to-be find a midwife they can trust to advise them during pregnancy and labour.

If –

If you can keep your head when all about you
Are losing theirs and blaming it on you,
If you can trust yourself when all men doubt you,
But make allowance for their doubting too;
If you can wait and not be tired by waiting,
Or being lied about don't deal in lies,
Or being hated, don't give way to hating,
And yet don't look too good, nor talk too wise:

If you can dream – and not make dreams your master;
If you can think – and not make thoughts your aim;
If you can meet with Triumph and Disaster
And treat those two impostors just the same;
If you can bear to hear the truth you've spoken
Twisted by knaves to make a trap for fools,
Or watch the things you gave your life to, broken,
And stoop and build 'em up with worn out tools:

If you can make a heap of all your winnings
And risk it on one turn of pitch-and-toss,
And lose, and start again at your beginnings
And never breathe a word about your loss;
If you can force your heart and nerve and sinew
To serve your turn long after they are gone,
And so hold on when there is nothing in you
Except the Will which says to them: "Hold on!"

If you can talk with crowds and keep your virtue,
Or walk with Kings – nor lose the common touch,
If neither foes nor loving friends can hurt you,
If all men count with you, but none too much;
If you can fill the unforgiving minute
With sixty seconds worth of distance run,
Yours is the Earth and everything that's in it,
And – which is more – you'll be a Man, my son!

Rudyard Kipling

(Or a mother, or a daughter, or a midwife or a good doctor.)

Preface

Never before have our homes been more comfortable, well heated and hygienic. Yet, despite the luxuries of modern life, we choose to leave the all embracing comfort and security of the home and to travel - sometimes for many miles, in the early stages of labour to have our babies in the alien environment of large hospitals!

During labour the father provides the mother with perhaps her only source of emotional support in an atmosphere of ruthless efficiency amongst complete strangers and amidst the technological paraphernalia of modern childbirth.

After the birth, the new family are allowed an hour to get to know each other in the recovery room before the father is pushed out into the cold to return alone to an empty house. He spends hours on the telephone telling the good news to all and sundry in a vain attempt to counteract his feelings of loneliness and isolation on what should be the happiest day of his life. His grandfather may have been denied a place at his father's actual birth, but he could at least share the magic moments of the first few hours of his son's life once the midwife had finished. The couple were then left in peace and both could contemplate the mysteries of parenthood and revel in the joys of a new life.

Today, back at the hospital, the mother is left by herself, with no one to share her feelings. She longs to take her new baby into bed with her and get to know this little bundle that she has felt for nine long months but has only just met. She does not dare to take the infant from his cot and cuddle him for fear that it might not be allowed. All too often the child has been taken away from her and put in another part of the hospital supposedly receiving special care while recovering from the shock of birth.

Is this the way we want to welcome our children into the world? Can it be right to subject ourselves to so much psychological violence at such a momentous point in our lives? Is this the best way to deal with childbirth in a civilised society?

How many obstetricians have seen the miracle of a joyful birth in the mother's own home? Perhaps one in a thousand. Most of them are doing their level best to ensure that such a thing can never happen again. They have deluded both themselves and us into thinking that childbirth in hospital is the only safe option for the 1990s and they will not be satisfied until they have drawn all labouring women into a hospital.

I hope to show just how misguided, physically dangerous and psychologically disastrous the present system is. Whether or not I succeed depends on your willingness to read this book with new eyes, to try to put aside any indoctrinated prejudices and see childbirth in a radically new light - to see it as an enriching experience to be welcomed joyfully rather than as a medical process to be endured for the sake of having children.

It would be unthinkable to present such a radical theory without also presenting the science on which the theory is based. Here I had a major problem, which to some extent I have been unable to overcome. The science is complicated, enveloping as it does many different scientific disciplines, each having its own body of knowledge and vocabulary to go with it. Some readers may find that they flounder helplessly in uncharted waters and find the science almost unreadable - I must admit that it seemed very nearly unwritable at times. If this is the case, skip the science and start at the chapter on labour. Come back to the science later on if, having read the rest, you are still sceptical.

But the professionals must not omit the science - it is presented especially for their benefit. Their very education and training has subjected them to so much brainwashing about "clinical childbirth" that they need as much science as possible to enable them to look at current practice afresh. It will take far more science to convince them that the concept that labour can be actively managed by professionals is as absurd as it is dangerous. Labour is women's work and "managed" by women's minds.

I could not cope with trying to be politically correct at the same time as translating scientific jargon into understandable English; when I say *man* the context usually dictates whether I mean the male of the species or the species itself. I usually refer to the foetus as *it*, its sex not usually being known until after the birth, and I usually refer to the baby as *he* simply to distinguish the baby from the mother.

There is so very little research into many of the aspects of childbirth dealt with in this book that it is all the more important to spread abroad what little information there is. This will enable the scientific and medical communities to take this research into account in their own work and practice. Mothers, more than anyone else, must become aware of the possible dangers of the modern way of birth, and be better informed before signing any consent forms. Much of the information we all need in order to become informed about birth is hidden away in learned journals, and some of it is available only in this book.

Sometimes I have wondered how I dare to criticise and question so many aspects of modern maternity practice but perhaps childbirth itself is an area where "Mother knows best."

Margaret Jowitt
Walford
November 1992

Childbirth Or Obstetrics?

"In 1972, A.C. Cochrane... rated obstetrics as the least scientifically based specialty within medical practice. My experience in reviewing the literature confirms that Cochrane's opinion is largely valid."

Derek Llewellyn-Jones, in *Fundamentals of Obstetrics and Gynaecology,* Faber and Faber, 1990.

The intention of this book is to put the real science into childbirth, to see through the medico-politics of clinical childbirth and to allow women to regain control of their own domain by letting them know how and why their bodies work in labour thus removing fear of the unknown. The science revealed in this book shows that, with very few exceptions, technology has no place in childbirth. The real science of childbirth teaches us that childbirth, like mothering, is an instinctive female art in which politics should play no part. Despite the apparent evidence to the contrary, most of the scientific evidence shows that, for the vast majority of women, home is the best and safest place in which to have a baby.

There are three main strands to my argument. The first is that we are better able to relax and heed our instincts in the comfort of our own homes – and our instincts are vitally important in the safe delivery of our infants; the second is that the unfamiliar environment of the hospital leads to higher secretion of stress hormones, all of which act to slow down labour; and the third is that our homes are physically removed from most of the sophisticated technology of modern birth and, if the machinery is not there, the temptation to make full use of it unnecessarily ceases to be a problem.

It is equally important that mother and baby should spend the first few days of life together at home with the father and the rest of the family; the hospital environment and hospital routines militate against maternal bonding and interfere with the natural consolidation of the new family.

Man, in his supreme arrogance, thinks that he can improve upon a superb engineering system that has taken millions of years of trial and error to evolve. Woman has lain down on the bed of childbirth like a lamb to the slaughter, has denied her own instincts and handed over responsibility for the survival of the baby she has carried within her for nine months to that half of mankind that knows least about it – the male of the species.

In no other aspect of childcare do we find men naturally better than women. Breast milk is far better for babies than man-made formula milk; most women seem to know instinctively how best to calm a crying baby and, even in these days of supposed equality of the sexes, childcare is still seen to be women's work. The vast majority of reception class teachers are female and we prefer a female baby-sitter to a male one. We all seem to accept quite happily that women are instinctively better than men at looking after babies. So why have women decided to ignore their instincts when instincts are most needed – in that most dangerous part of a baby's life, its birth? Why also do we so mistrust our maternal instincts after the birth and stay in hospital being taught how to look after a new born baby? Are we, the most intelligent of animals, naturally inept at childcare?

There is no doubt that most professionals believe this to be the case. Over the last century or so there has been an enormously successful propaganda campaign that has proceeded almost unnoticed by the general public, so skilful has been its execution. We have handed over responsibility for our children's birth to obstetricians. Even midwives now work predominantly under obstetricians and many have lost vital skills and experience in caring for labouring women. Midwives are fighting to retain their professional autonomy as independent practitioners responsible for normal birth. Today hospital-based medicine has very nearly achieved its aim of ensuring that all babies are born in consultant maternity units, so-called centres of excellence – or at least in cars or ambulances on the way there!

This book is an attempt to turn the tide before it is too late. I sympathise with King Canute. I know just how he felt with the sea gently lapping round his toes, faced with a great flood of water threatening to drag him under. But there are three main differences between us. He knew that he could not turn the tide, whereas I very much hope that I can. He was being urged by his sycophantic followers to stem the forces of nature, whereas I am trying to stem the forces of man. He was risking only his own life whereas I am attempting to improve and enrich the lives of all our unborn children and their families by showing that nature, when given the chance, does a far better job than meddlesome man.

I can almost hear the great sighs of relief from the hidebound obstetrical establishment – yet another cranky Green book by a nature freak; nothing to upset the apple-cart here. I shall play devil's advocate for a while and see if I can nudge the obstetricians out of their complacency. I'll give them the benefit of the first word:

Aha, says my caricature of an obstetrician of the old school, *Nature is red in tooth and claw. If anything goes wrong with a natural birth the baby dies, often killing its mother in the process. Just think how high the mortality rates were before our profession started to improve on nature.*

How very true, say I. For million of years Nature has been improving on the mechanism of childbirth in the most brutal way possible – by killing her mistakes. There were no forceps deliveries and caesarean sections to rescue women who failed to deliver naturally. The childbirth genes of those women and children were weeded out by the forces of natural selection. On the other hand, obstetricians have been attempting to improve on Nature for only a few hundred years. The first few decades of hospital childbirth actually worsened

14

women's lot by exposing hundreds of women to the risk of puerperal fever. Do you seriously believe that your profession has made such enormous strides in the short time since then?

Medicine has made enormous leaps since those early days. Besides, nature cares not one iota whether an individual lives or dies in childbed.

Hospital-based obstetrics doesn't treat women as individuals, many women complain of being treated like cattle.

Nature is concerned only with the survival of genetic material. Nature wants to weed out bad specimens. We want to save everyone.

Point taken, but I am not convinced that your motives are entirely altruistic. Don't you rather enjoy having so much control over the perpetuation of the species? Don't you revel in your position as a god at the top of the hierarchy? The income isn't bad is it? Though you might earn more in the USA. It must give your ego a kick having all those women queuing up for hours to see you every day and hanging on to your every word.

We reach our position after many years of hard work, studying through the night, up at all hours, sacrificing family life ourselves for the sake of our patients. It is only right that we should be well rewarded as a result.

Perhaps the sacrifice of family life is the reason why so few women doctors are able to go into obstetrics, which has always seemed to me to be rather odd. After all, only women can have personal experience of childbirth.

Personal experience counts for very little, our experience comes from many years of learning about the many problems that accompany parturition and treating hundreds of women in labour. We can learn far more quickly than nature. The blind forces of natural selection work very slowly but we can share our experience and learn from our mistakes in the time it takes to make a phone call or to publish an article in a journal.

Quite so, but does it really make any difference to the way you practice? It took years and years of research findings before routine enemas and shaving of pubic hair were abandoned.

Think instead of all the advances in pain relief in the last twenty years. Nature makes women suffer. We can offer them the benefits of modern pain relief.

Women labouring at home need hardly any pain relief. Shouldn't research be directed at finding out what causes pain instead of perpetuating the practice of removing pain artificially? Mothers have sold their birthright for that mess of pottage known as pain relief. It has been used as a carrot to lure them into hospital. Throughout pregnancy we are constantly told to avoid all unnecessary drugs, then at the most dangerous time of all, for both mother and baby, we get stuffed full with them.

In this day and age women have a right to pain relief. Natural childbirth is all very well and we do our best to accommodate the mother's wishes but, when it comes down to it, we have two patients on our hands, the mother and the baby. Sometimes we have to overrule the mother's wishes and do what is best for the baby – and hospital is the place for that. You have only to look at how maternal and neonatal mortality rates have fallen as we have managed to find hospital beds for all women in order to see the strength of the argument against home birth.

I see, so babies born at home are more likely to die are they? According to recent statistics, a Dutch mother delivered by a consultant in hospital is 18 times more likely to lose her baby as one delivered by a midwife at home.

Dutch women are made differently and of course, Dutch consultants get all the high risk patients, which rather distorts the figures. Modern antenatal care can anticipate and prevent many problems.

I thought that you could only predict about half potential problems in labour before the event. Presumably half the home birth Dutch women had unforeseen problems as well.

It really is most unwise not to seek medical supervision during pregnancy so that problems can be foreseen and dealt with appropriately. We can do so much more today than we could fifty years ago.

I agree that antenatal care can be useful but I'm talking about labour itself. I've heard that even British statistics show no increased risk for a home or GP unit delivery.

That's only a result of better selection of high risk patients. Home birth is dangerous and should be outlawed. GP units are an anachronism in this day and age. All women should have access to the most up-to-date obstetrical practice. Moreover, all newborn babies should be born in a place where first-rate paediatric services are available. It's all very well for a mother to risk her own life but to submit her child to the risks of a home birth is scandalous.

The statistics actually show a reduced risk both in GP units and at home for mother and baby alike, despite the absence of paediatric services.

Statistics don't prove anything, besides, I'd be more inclined to believe the figures if that work had been done by a man. Women have a vested interest is these things. We have to save them from their female whims. Besides, we have improved things a lot since then. Nowadays we are much more relaxed – most women bring their husbands in with them, you know, we encourage it. They can look after their wife's emotional needs while we can get on with the real work. I shouldn't bother your head with statistics, my dear, childbirth is safer in 1992 than it has ever been.

Could it be stress hormones that interfere with labour in hospital? Hospital is a very stressful place for ordinary people. Doesn't adrenaline stop contractions?

Adrenaline goes up every time the telephone rings, we can't do anything about that.

What about ß-endorphin (beta-endorphin)? Scientists have discovered a lot about ß-endorphin and reproduction recently.

ß-endorphin... Yes. That's there to relieve the pain.

It also stops smooth muscle contracting.

Does it indeed? I shouldn't worry too much about the hormones, my dear. Stress is a funny sort of thing. It has all sorts of unexpected side effects. What is stress anyway? Psychologists should try to find out if hospital childbirth actually is stressful before jumping to wild unsubstantiated conclusions about stress hormones in labour. Most women are relieved by the knowledge that they are giving birth in the safety of hospital with all the facilities there should something go wrong. Indeed, we obstetricians can and do take women's stress on ourselves. We have quite enough stress already. I wouldn't want to add to my own stress by allowing home deliveries. We're trying to make hospitals more like home now. We don't induce unless we have to and we let women do what they want for the first stage of labour. The days of stirrup deliveries are long past.

Perhaps hospitals are a little more like home than they were ten years ago. But I'd still do anything to avoid a hospital birth and, given the ambivalent figures, I still don't see why you have to discourage home birth quite so vehemently.

I'm afraid it's the women's own fault. They sue us if anything goes wrong. Childbirth is still a risky business so we have to put mothers in hospital where we can keep an eye on them, just in case'.

You could get people wanting home births to sign a disclaimer saying that they had acted against medical advice.

It wouldn't wash, my dear, it wouldn't carry any legal weight. We are the professionals and the law expects us to act accordingly. No. I'm afraid you have no one but yourselves to blame. Parents expect a perfect result and we have to do all we can to achieve it for them, but birth is still the most dangerous time of a baby's life, and we are going to lose some of them whatever we do – and then the parents look around for someone to sue. We have to do everything we can so the lawyers can't prove we missed something and were negligent. You've brought it on yourselves, you know.

I'm having my baby at home anyway. The Queen had her babies at home.

The Queen had the advantage of a fully equipped operating theatre downstairs should she have needed it. If you were the Queen I'd let you have your baby at home. But you're not and if you decide to have a home delivery I'll wash my hands of you.

We seem to have come a long way from discussing nature.

17

We really can't leave things all to nature these days, whatever the Greens may say. We give nature a helping hand and achieve far better results. Yes, I'm glad to say that hospital childbirth is here to stay and the sooner all women see sense the better. Now, if you will excuse me, I really am far too busy to talk to you any more. It's Friday morning and I've six women to deliver today if I am to have a weekend to myself.

Thank you for being so generous with your time. Sorry to have bothered you.

Really, if people want to become obstetricians they should realise that nature doesn't recognise weekends and Bank Holidays... And why am I apologising for wasting his time... Surely it's part of his job to reassure women with his superior knowledge... It's in his own interests to maintain the status quo...

He underestimates my intelligence but then he is used to seeing women as wombs on legs and probably doesn't realise that women have brains. Perhaps I have been too hard on him, after all he's only doing his job and if he sincerely believes that childbirth is safer in hospital then he is right to try and stop me in my tracks. He doesn't have to argue as strongly as I do, he has the establishment on his side. Look how the establishment quashed the House of Commons Select Committee that came out in favour of home births. The Government sacked the chairman. There must be a huge vested interest somewhere. He doesn't really have much to worry about. Women have been trying for years to reclaim childbirth and look what they have achieved so far: wallpaper in the first stage room, and birth plans not worth the paper they are written on. Mere window dressing! When are we going to be allowed to decide where and when to give birth to our own babies? Whose babies are they?

At first sight the statistical evidence seems to prove the doctor right and me wrong. However, there are "lies, damned lies and statistics." Statistics can be made to prove anything if you ask the wrong questions or if you omit relevant parameters from your analysis. Statistics have indeed shown a strong correlation between the rise in hospital births and the decrease in mortality figures for both mothers and babies in this century. However, this correlation is a coincidence – the association can be more than accounted for by other factors. When re-analysed, the existing data on birth tell a very different story than that related by the medical establishment. Marjorie Tew has produced an excellent reanalysis of the existing statistics in her book *Safer Childbirth* (Chapman and Hall, 1990). Despite having been an advocate of home birth for many years I still found it hard to believe that I had safety on my side as well as common sense and humanity. I believe with her that the statistics show that we ignore nature at our peril and that the mortality figures could be reduced even further if we listened to nature's advice. Doctors are lowering the mortality figures artificially at the moment by terminating many pregnancies that would otherwise end in the death of the child, but even today the UK

18

stillbirth rate is one of the highest in Western Europe. There is a long way to go.

Nature alone can select the best genes for the job of childbirth; we have to work on the material that nature provides. Very occasionally doctors can counteract the effects of genetic failure, for example by providing an antidote to Rhesus iso-immunisation which can result in blue babies. More often they decide to weed out nature's errors by so-called therapeutic abortion. Where individual women fail to achieve their genetic potential and have a poor physique for childbearing, doctors can tinker with the mechanics of the body and, doubtless, many lives have been saved that way, though fewer in recent years since most women are far better fed in childhood and consequently healthier than once they were.

However, these very successes have made doctors arrogant enough to think that they can do better than nature all the time and, in their arrogance, they have tinkered too long and too much. They put lives at risk through far too many medical and surgical procedures, from oxytocin drips to caesarean sections, which research has shown to be unnecessary and even harmful at times. One obstetrician has stated that there are no contraindications to a caesarean section, despite very clear evidence to the contrary regarding its after effects on both mother and baby.

The obstetrician's work is all but finished after the child's delivery but the parents' work has only just begun. Who is responsible for bringing babies into the world? Is it the obstetrician who declares a job finished once a healthy baby is extricated from a healthy mother? Or is it the parents, the people who take the responsibility of a family upon themselves?

Giving responsibility for birth itself to the NHS, acting on behalf of the State, teaches parents straightaway that the State is responsible for their children. Are we right to blame parents of troublesome teenagers caught joyriding for lack of parental control and lack of responsibility for their badly behaving offspring? If society has denied parents responsibility and control at the birth of those children, society must take the blame for the consequences. The rise in hospital birth has also coincided with rising divorce rates, rising delinquency, rising tranquillizer prescriptions, falling moral values and even falling church attendance. Birth is a spiritual experience as well as a physiological event. Is hospital childbirth destroying man's very soul?

If hospital childbirth is so dangerous, how have women been lured into the trap of thinking that childbirth on the male medical model is so good? Women were enticed into hospital by promises of pain relief and easy labours. But the so-called pain of childbirth was invented by civilisation and reinforced by men. Even the Bible was pressed into the task of fuelling the myth of unavoidably painful childbirth. The authorised version of Genesis, chapter 3, verse 16, reads: "In sorrow shalt thou bring forth children." Sorrow is totally alien to my own experience of childbirth. In joy I brought forth my children. The Revised Standard Version of 1952 is even worse – "I will greatly multiply your pain in childbearing; in pain you shall bring forth children."

However, it is man rather than God who has greatly multiplied our pain in childbearing. The words sorrow and pain are mischievous mistranslations; the same Hebrew word is translated as labour or toil elsewhere in the Bible. I have no quarrel with that – childbirth is certainly hard labour but, as it says in Proverbs, "In all labour there is profit", and what greater profit than the birth of a child?

The sorrow of modern childbirth is that the joy of birth has been confiscated and parents have been given a secondary role to play. Parents and children have become mere pawns in NHS politics. NHS politics are largely determined by consultants. The consultant has become the most important person on the scene, ousting both the mother and her baby from their rightful place. A modern picture of the Madonna and Christ Child would have to have a picture of the Archangel Gabriel dressed in a white coat hovering discreetly in the background to take the credit. It adds insult to injury to be told that medical childbirth is for our own good, and we are doubly insulted when we discover that unnecessary intervention puts mothers, babies and family life at risk. Friday afternoon caesarean sections benefit only the consultant and the hospital routine; the health of mother and baby come a poor third and fourth; the father is virtually ignored.

Yet despite the growing body of evidence against hospital childbirth, most people are still convinced of its safety. Women were enticed into hospital with the promise of pain relief but received more of what had caused the pain in the first place – drugs and physical confinement. Once there, they were controlled by dire threats of what would go wrong if they were bad patients and did not do as they were told. Even worse trouble was predicted for anyone who wanted to have her baby at home. Modern women's fears of pain and danger are reinforced by the medical model of childbirth and the only advantages are a few days break from cooking and childcare, and the camaraderie of fellow inmates.

Today, hardly anyone dares even to ask for a home confinement, let alone resist nine months of constant anti-home birth propaganda. However, research has shown that women labouring at home not only feel less pain, but also have a far more positive experience of birth and are far less likely to have complications during labour or postnatal depression. They are also more successful in establishing breastfeeding. Encouraging home birth could save vast amounts of money. The establishment has avoided making direct comparisons of costs but estimates have varied between £100 and £300 per day for hospital confinement. Every pound spent on keeping healthy mothers and babies in hospital could be spent on far better things. New mothers could even have a small allowance to help pay someone to help with the housework while recovering from the birth and getting to know the new baby.

An eminent obstetrician has spoken of "wicked women with their malicious lying tongues" referring to the horror stories many women have to tell about their labours. Most of those horror stories now tell of insensitive and inhuman treatment at the hands of hospital staff. I have heard and read numerous accounts of women being coerced into treatment they did not want; of their partners being won over by the medical staff in efforts to get women to change their minds – given dire threats of the risks of death to mother and baby if the mother refused to comply with advice. To whom do the lying and malicious tongues now belong?

The doctors have done their best to foster dependence on themselves. One notable exception was Dr. Grantly Dick-Read, a London GP who, in his book *Childbirth Without Fear*, quotes the words of a working class woman spoken after her baby was born at home: "It didn't hurt. It wasn't meant to, was it Doctor?" Her rhetorical question spurred Dick-Read on to investigate the pain of childbirth. His fear-tension-pain explanation of pain in childbirth led to the formation of the Natural Childbirth Association (later to become the National Childbirth Trust and later still, and how shamefully, to cut out all references to his teaching from their literature, Jenny Kitzinger, 1990). I bought my copy of his book from the for sale shelves of Winchester public library where I also found Sheila Kitzinger's book *Birth at Home* (published in 1979 and discarded in about 1987). The medical propaganda has been so sucessful that even librarians are censoring our reading material (or perhaps the books were slung out because Winchester women refused to believe that any woman could have her baby at home without fear, and so left the books on the shelf for too long?). Dick-Read received very shabby treatment from the women he was trying to help and the result has been that, fifty years later, they continue to receive shabby treatment from his less enlightened colleagues.

Childbirth Without Fear and *Birth at Home* started me on the long road to this book. They gave me the chance to have two of my three children happily at home. When I rang *The Times* to place a birth announcement on the day my son was born, the girl on the phone found it hard to believe that birth could be happy. It makes me intensely sad that most women are denied that experience and it makes me hopping mad that I have been hoodwinked by the medical profession into doubting that the safest possible place for most children to be born is in their own home.

I had originally assumed the benefits of home delivery to be mainly psychological and thought that the psychological benefits would outweigh the medical risks. This is indeed the case, but I then discovered that hospital birth actually *increases* the medical risks and was greatly alarmed. I have been moved to tears at the accounts of the risks and dangers labouring women have been exposed to in the name of medical knowledge while being denied the joy of delivering their children in the safety and comfort of their own home. I applied to my old university to do some research myself only to find that many people had done it before me and had already found the results I expected to find. Yet still the medical establishment wants to retain control of childbirth and severely disciplines dissenting midwives and even obstetricians within its own ranks.

While awaiting permission to start a small study comparing the outcome of labours at home and in hospital, I started to look at the role of stress hormones in labour. If women labouring at home really need less pain relief and birth is actually safer at home, then the mind must play a larger role in labour than has previously been thought. The standard explanation is that the actual pain is the same in both places, it is only women's ability to cope with pain that varies. I disagree having had both painfree and painful labour contractions. *The theoretical underpinning for the statistical and anecdotal evidence for the better quality of home births become abundantly clear once the hormonal control of labour is understood.*

We must turn the tide and return to a balanced view of childbirth as soon as possible. Already it is too late for most women today. It will take many years to undo the effects of the obstetricians' propaganda. They have managed to convince nearly everyone that hospital birth is the only safe option. Many women will just not be prepared to take the so-called risk of a home birth against such powerful brainwashing so, for the time being, most of us will have to put up with the hospital service, although this could be improved beyond recognition.

I have to convince you that hospital birth is dangerous, not only because obstetricians are too quick to intervene but also because the mere act of going to hospital slows down labour, leads to pain and often the dreaded intervention – oxytocin drips, forceps and caesarean sections. Moreover, postnatal hospital care condemns countless mothers and children to life-long emotional stress by interfering with the mother/child bond. Hospital birth is dangerous in itself before any meddlesome midwifery confounds the situation. How am I to convince not only women themselves but also their husbands, midwives, GPs and obstetricians? I will eschew anecdotal evidence as much as possible since this is despised in our great age of science. I will proceed by turning the question on its head. Instead of asking why childbirth is such an ordeal, I will try to find out what Nature intended and why it has gone wrong.

Perhaps in fifty years time the medical history books will record with incredulity that in the late twentieth century hospital childbirth became the rule not the exception. They will note that the perinatal mortality rate could have fallen to 1 or 2 in 1000 instead of 6 in 1000 decades sooner than it did. They will throw up their hands in horror at the high levels of brain-damaged babies and depressed mothers. Perhaps social historians will agree with me that many of the ills of modern society resulted from the inappropriate twentieth century practice of treating labouring women as ignorant and incompetent fools. I look forward to the days when the tables will be turned and we give all women the chance to have their babies happily at home.

THE SCIENCE

OF

CHILDBIRTH

1   Evolution

Natura non facit saltum (Nature does not make jumps)

Darwin

In the last chapter I seemed to make the sweeping assumption that "Nature knows best". Of course nature does not *know* anything. Nature just is. Before I go any further you need to know my working definition of nature which is the same as most other people's definition. I do not regard nature as a sort of latter-day god. I use the word nature in its strictest scientific sense.

"Mother Nature" was a term invented by man to account for phenomena over which he had no control. (It is ironical to note, however, that he made her feminine). Man personalised nature because it made him better able to think about the things he observed around him. In most early cultures natural phenomena were given human personalities. Ra represented the sun for the ancient Egyptians and Thor personified thunder in Norse mythology. But it was easy to fall into the trap of endowing the concept itself with human attributes. Man observed causes and effects in his surroundings and mistakenly gave nature the human attribute of purposefulness. Speaking scientifically, nature has no purpose at all. It is a convenient shorthand for distinguishing between that which is man made and that which is not. *Natural* describes things that are not under man's conscious control. With this definition we can describe, for example, the nature/nurture controversy as a struggle between genetic determinism on the one hand and man's interventions on the other.

The whole of this book is concerned with the level of man's interventions (both as direct interference and as indirect consequences of civilisation) in a genetically programmed event – childbirth – and in genetically programmed behaviour – mothering. Having forestalled, I hope, some justifiable criticism of the view that Nature knows best, I can now proceed with the main thesis of this chapter which is that the blind process of natural selection has produced a potentially highly efficient mechanism for childbirth.

Natural selection has done a first rate job of colonising the earth with *Homo sapiens* (and, unfortunately, in giving Western man domination over the world's flora and fauna). This task was more or less complete well before doctors arrived on the scene. Insofar as we are all here, natural selection succeeded in propagating our ancestors' genes without the aid of medical technology until the advent of doctors. There may well have been elements of unnatural selection since then so, for the moment, I will concentrate on the obstetric history of mankind until the dawn of civilisation.

No doubt there will be some who argue that all I have done is to exchange King Log for King Stork – that natural selection is as incompetent as nature where human childbirth is concerned. Certainly evolution paints a grim picture of natural selection – a crude, cruel and ruthless perpetrator of the most heinous crimes: matricide, fratricide and genocide. For many people evolution is nothing more than an interesting theory accounting for the fossil record. The only part of the theory seen to have any relevance today is the concept of extinction, which we see as a threat to our modern world; we tend to see evolution as a negative process – the elimination of unsuccessful species. But evolution is better seen as a positive force that accounts for all existing life on earth. All present life forms are the result of successive and successful adaptations to previous life forms, resulting in the rich diversity of living organisms that we see today. It is this aspect of evolution that is central to my argument.

Darwin's theory of evolution states that different forms of life have evolved over millions of years through *natural selection*, the selective weeding out of individuals that failed to thrive and reproduce and of species that failed to adapt to a changing environment, or failed to produce enough offspring to ensure the continuation of their line. Richard Dawkins in his book *The Selfish Gene* suggests that the survival and reproduction of the gene itself is even more pertinent to evolution, a body is merely a gene survival and reproduction machine. The organism provides a benign environment for the propagation of genes and it acts as a buffer between the gene and the outside world. The survival of an organism depends on its physical characteristics and these depend on the organism's genes and its physical environment. Different genes affect survival and reproduction rates differently in different environments. A useful gene for a particular organism in a particular environment gets copied into more individuals than a useless or harmful one; a gene that aids survival and reproduction will tend to spread through the population; a gene that aids survival of the individual while reducing its chances of reproduction is likely to spread much more slowly – if at all. Natural selection ensures that good genes get copied, reproduced, into more bodies than bad genes. When understood at the level of the gene, the power of natural selection appears all the more compelling and relentless.

The alternative phrase, *survival of the fittest*, glosses over the central role played by reproduction. Reproduction is the be-all-and-end-all of evolutionary theory; it is the yardstick by which survival is ultimately measured. However well individuals or genes survived in one lifetime, unless they also reproduced successfully, they were on the road to extinction. Before we start to look at what has gone wrong with human reproduction it would seem eminently sensible to look at what has gone right with it.

The heredity/environment or nature/nurture controversy rages as much in this book as in other fields. Is dangerous childbirth part of man's genetic heritage or do environmental factors play a larger role than has been suspected hitherto? Have women in past ages failed to achieve their genetic potential and is modern Western woman closer to the genetic ideal? If so, why is childbirth still painful and dangerous?

DNA – a recipe for life

Practically all living cells contain a complete set of instructions written in the chemical code of DNA (deoxyribonucleic acid), a set of genes, for replicating not just themselves, but the organism as a whole. Theoretically it would be possible to look at the DNA in the nucleus of a cell and describe the life form it belonged to down to the last detail. Sets of genes determine the *genotype*. But this theoretical possibility belongs in the realms of science fiction, we have 100,000 genes, each of which will have more than one physical effect. Moreover, the actual organism, the *phenotype*, depends as much upon the environment in which it matured and inhabits. For example, the genotype could never predict an amputated limb or even actual height. It could perhaps predict *potential* height but height *actually achieved* would depend on availability of environmental necessities such as food, oxygen and sunlight. Environmental factors decide how the DNA recipe is to be transcribed into life. Nurture is part of nature itself.

Genes

Genes are snippets of heritable information on how to make a particular attribute or function of a body – from eye colour, colour perception, blood group and blood clotting ability to such esoteric functions as the ability to waggle one's ears – an inherited party trick. Genes are chemical templates for making amino acids, the building blocks of proteins which are themselves the building blocks of life. The layman thinks of protein as meat, but many other constituents of the body are proteins as well, for example enzymes and some hormones, both of which are catalysts for changes in cell function.

In sexually reproducing organisms genes come in pairs, one inherited from the female and one from the male, but only one is used for making the body. For the vast majority of traits the genes inherited from the mother and father will be the same. Our differences are as nothing compared to our similarities. Indeed we share 99% of our genes with chimpanzees. But for certain traits there may be a choice between two different genes, for example, blue eyes or brown eyes and the strongest gene, the dominant gene, wins the fight for inclusion in the body. Weaker genes, recessive genes, will be expressed in the body only when DNA inherited from both mother and father lacks the stronger one. Because a double set of genes is carried, twice the amount of genetic material than is strictly necessary is carried forward to the next generation. Although recessive genes may not be expressed they can still pass down the generations.

Sexual reproduction increased the rate of evolutionary change by providing a means of shuffling genetic material about from generation to generation.

Mutations

DNA reproduces itself all the time as genes are translated into proteins, and cells divide to form new cells – growth and repair of the individual body – but it can reproduce over evolutionary time by putting copies of itself into eggs and sperm which then unite to form a new body or gene survival machine. DNA is extremely good at making copies of itself but very occasionally the copying goes wrong – it makes a mistake just once in every 10,000 transcriptions. Radiation from medical X-rays, from the sun and from nuclear accidents causes gene transcription mistakes. The incidence of skin cancer will increase as the ozone layer thins and becomes less effective at screening out harmful radiation. Ironically, breast cancer may be increased by routine X-ray screening. There is mounting evidence that men working in the nuclear industries produce mutated sperm. The effects on female reproduction will take longer to ascertain because a woman is born with her full quota of hereditary DNA – her eggs – whereas men manufacture new sperm. There will be a twenty-year delay between noticing genetic accidents caused by mutated DNA in sperm and finding genetic accidents caused by mutated DNA in ova.

Mutations are caused by tiny changes in a gene making it produce a slightly different protein. Changes in cell function can have far reaching effects. Cancers are caused by mutations increasing rate of cell division in non-hereditary cells. They start by a change in one cell but can spread to affect different cells in other parts of the body. Most of the time the body's immune system notices such changes and kills the mutating cell but if the immune system is suppressed by stress hormones the mutation may spread and a cancer forms.

A single change in a protein caused by a mutant gene in an egg or a sperm, carriers of hereditary DNA, can have similarly far reaching effects on body function in the developing embryo. Most such changes are as lethal as cancer can be but, just occasionally, a mutation in egg or sperm DNA turns out to be beneficial and bodies carrying the new gene survive and reproduce more than bodies carrying the old one.

Most mutations are lethal – the pregnancy is likely to miscarry spontaneously (60% of miscarriages are thought to be owed to a defective foetus) or the child is stillborn, or born with a genetic defect. However, some mutants do survive and have offspring and, over evolutionary time, mutant genes can spread throughout a population, aided and abetted by sexual reproduction which shuffles genes around forming unique individuals every time (apart from identical twins who share all their genes because they develop from the same fertilised egg).

When seen from the perspective of a single lifetime, or even just a couple of centuries (in man whose life cycle is very long compared to less complicated species) it does not seem possible that beneficial mutations could occur often enough to have a major effect on the development of a species. However, all life on earth evolved from the very first bit of DNA that learnt how to copy itself. Evolution is powerful enough to explain the differences between ants and elephants, both of which have the common ancestor of the first bit of DNA. "I trace my ancestry to a protoplasmal primordial atomic globule," says Pooh Bah in Gilbert and Sullivan's The Mikado.

When seen over evolutionary time, measured in millions of years and billions of generations, good mutations become commonplace and the results are there for all to see in the fossil record.

Constraints on natural selection

Before I start to outline the evolution of man with particular reference to reproduction I must put in a cautionary note for myself as much as for my readers. We must not fall into the trap of thinking that natural selection has provided the best solution to all problems. Natural selection can only work with the genes that exist in the gene pool together with the odd mutation. Man is a placental mammal and a woman produces a child by nourishing her foetus *in utero* for nine months, delivering a live infant, feeding it milk and nurturing it until it reaches the point where it can fend for itself in the world. We may wish that natural selection had chosen some other way of producing children, and given us less work to do in rearing them, but nature cannot go back to the drawing board and design a different birthing process for the convenience of modern woman or her doctor who might prefer a zip fastening womb. Nature is limited to making improvements to existing mechanisms.

Nature can also make genetic mistakes in individuals. In a very few instances, by knowing the particular protein affected by a defective gene, man can limit its ill effects. People with haemophilia can be given the missing protein, factor VIII. Scientists are closer to finding a genetically engineered cure for cystic fibrosis and hope to be able to insert the missing gene into bone marrow (which is a factory for making many different proteins). We know that Down's syndrome is caused by an extraneous chunk of DNA but can do nothing to cure it.

Our genetic recipe, or *genotype*, usually dictates instructions for making an ideal human being. But for the recipe to be translated into an ideal *phenotype*, the environment must supply exactly the right ingredients in exactly the right quantities at each stage of maturation from the very first division of the fertilised egg to the grave itself. We are only too aware of how often the social environment fails to supply the right ingredients for optimum educational achievement, and we are becoming ever more aware of how the physical environment exerts its effect on our physical development. The richer classes are healthier than the poorest.

Earlier this century the state became aware of the link between childhood nutrition and the desired end result, a strong healthy adult. Wanting to improve the physical quality of its population it instituted the school meals service. Twenty years later maternal mortality in childbirth started to fall dramatically. Similarly, during the Second World War and with the coming of the Welfare State the health authorities started to look after pregnant women and babies better, providing orange juice and Marmite. Infant mortality fell dramatically. These physical improvements enabled more of us to follow our genetic recipe more closely. The policy of taking away NHS orange juice and school meals, and transferring resources into high-tech birth is a policy of madness and accounts for the increasing problems in the health of the poorer members of our society. There has always been a statistical correlation between income and health - including perinatal mortality - and high-tech medicine treats the effects rather than preventing problems in the first place. However, most of us are probably nearer our genetic ideal than ever before, so why is childbirth still painful and dangerous?

Our genetic recipe dictates instructions for efficient childbirth - it has to. Reproduction is the lynchpin of gene survival which depends on the survival of a healthy mother and child. When things go wrong the cause is still far more likely to be in our environment than in our genes. Is there anything else in our environment that might give a clue to the cause? Perhaps civilisation itself is responsible for the remaining problems of human childbirth. But let us put environmental factors aside for the moment and try to determine how the genetic recipe for childbirth evolved.

Evolution of Man

The evolution of man started when life first appeared on earth. Man gradually accumulated his genetic make up one step at a time over billions of years and millions of generations. The very beginning of this journey started about three thousand million years ago when the first primitive organism capable of making copies of itself arose out of the primaeval soup. However, the very earliest years need not concern us. We can start the story with the emergence of the mammals, a mere 180 million years ago, or perhaps 140 million years earlier than that - an estimate of how long it took for the mammal class to become differentiated from their reptilian vertebrate cousins. The most significant legacy from the vertebrates was the foundation of the hormone system which offered a means of controlling bodily functions relative to the environment and prepared the path for a closer linkage between body and mind, so important in instinctive behaviour.

Mammals

Mammals first emerged during the Cretaceous age when dinosaurs still roamed the earth. The mammals were warm-blooded and, being able to regulate their body temperature, could inhabit places out of reach of the cold-blooded reptiles. They were small, probably nocturnal, and kept out of the way of the dinosaurs. The dinosaurs became extinct, perhaps because of a natural catastrophe or perhaps because of over-specialisation (where a species has adapted to suit one particular environment so well that it has lost the ability to adapt to changes in that environment). At this stage mammals took the place of the large reptiles and quickly came to dominate the evolutionary landscape. Mammals did well for four reasons. First, each species found and exploited a previously unused environmental niche and so had fewer competitors; second, they were able to find and exploit niches in colder places because of a newly found ability to control their body temperature; third, their increased brain size made individuals better able learn to adapt to their environment day by day; and fourth they learnt to build nests - to manipulate the environment itself so that it suited their needs better.

The dinosaurs are usually seen as little more than huge, lumbering robots propelled by innate reflex actions, but mammals developed the ability to learn. Their larger brains could make new associations by wiring up new pathways in the brain. As the need arose, they could wire up innate reflex responses into patterns of learned instinctive behaviour. For example, they could learn to associate vibrations of the ground with the arrival of a predatory dinosaur. The first few times they felt the vibrations they would ignore them and run for cover only when they saw the predator, escaping death by the skin of their teeth, but eventually they learned to hide as soon as the ground started to vibrate.

Innate reflex responses still determined the physiological working of their bodies and much of their behaviour, but a new capacity to profit from past experience was introduced - intelligence. These qualitatively different brains made mammals better at exploiting their environments, and their brains also became bigger as mammals inheriting larger brain capacity had a greater ability to learn from their mistakes and consequently increased their chances of survival and reproduction. In their play infant mammals exercise their minds - they learn appropriate responses to perceptual stimuli that may increase their chance of survival when they attain adulthood, when their mother is no longer there to watch over them.

A larger brain also meant that there were more brain cells available to spend on, for example, better vision - to see one's prey or predator before it saw you. Mammals became specialists in different fields. Some have become extinct in the same way that the dinosaurs did when the environment changed drastically, but there is still an enormous variety of mammals adapted to suit all sorts of different environments and climates in land, sea and air.

Evolution of mammalian reproduction
Reproduction is the very way by which the class of mammals is named. Females have mammary glands to suckle their young. The first mammals took an enormous evolutionary gamble in deciding to develop a new mode of reproduction. They put more and more responsibility on to the female for the survival of the young. Most other forms of life use the safety in numbers principle and are profligate with their seed, laying many eggs, producing vast numbers of potential beings in the hope that enough will survive to propagate the species. However, female mammals produce just a few eggs at a time and give their offspring the best start in life by giving each child individual attention both while still in the womb, and after birth through the provision of milk. This method of reproduction is very expensive in terms of energy costs to the female; she invests an enormous amount of effort into rearing just a few young. Modern woman takes this principle to the extreme and puts her reproductive effort into producing just a handful of offspring in a lifetime of three-score years and ten. Lower orders of animals are profligate with their eggs, and, indeed, male mammals are profligate with their sperm, producing millions of sperm at each ejaculation, but the female has a relatively small number of chances to pass on her genes. Nurture is thus part of nature for the female mammal; unless she nurtures her young she will die childless.

The selection pressures for birthing baby mammals - and surviving the

31

experience – are very strong. If a female dies giving birth she cannot pass on her genes to any further offspring and, deprived of its natural food supply, the offspring will also die. If her child dies at birth, or indeed at any time up to the age of reproduction, he will not pass on his (and his mother's) genes. Any gene that tended to make childbirth more difficult would become rare in the population whereas any gene that increased the chances of bearing a child and raising him to reproductive age would tend to become more common.

There must be very many genes that have some effect on childbirth since it is such a complex event: genes affecting physique, reproductive apparatus, hormones, age of menarche, mothering behaviour and temperament, to name but the most obvious. For each possible choice, creatures possessing the better gene would be more likely to produce more offspring who themselves would produce more offspring until the detrimental genes would tend to be progressively wiped out.

The mammalian reproductive system is very good at adapting species to fit environments. Giving mothers more and more direct control over the fate of their eggs – giving birth to live infants and feeding them with purpose-made mother's milk – more than compensated for the smaller quantity of eggs fertilised. We see the strength of the selection forces for evolution of maternal behaviour. Young mammals in the wild quite simply could not survive without an adequate mother. Maternal behaviour was far too important to leave to chance – it had to be inherited. And from small beginnings evolved creatures able to survive in the Arctic or the tropics, creatures as diverse as whales and bats, mice and men.

The primates

Man's tree-dwelling ancestors, the first primates, appeared about 70 million years ago and took their first tentative steps on *terra firma* 20 million years ago. Other mammals specialised in various physical skills such as acute hearing, sharp vision, and running fast (to avoid death or hunt dinner) but the primates eventually specialised in brain power itself and, by virtue of their increased ability to learn from experience, became the most adaptable of the mammals. Primates specialised in intelligence itself. Living in trees, they had few predators. They could spend more time learning how to exploit their environment. The primate brain became progressively larger and gradually assumed a sponge-like capacity for absorbing and encoding new experiences. These larger brains had the capacity to observe and record cause and effect, and thus to adapt their owner's behaviour to suit circumstances. Infants spent a long time fashioning their instinctive behaviour to suit their particular environment; they could afford to make more mistakes as their mother was constantly looking after them and prepared to rush to their rescue.

Life in the trees required new skills. These first primates became adapted to jumping from branch to branch; they developed grasping limbs, with fingers and toes becoming more useful, particularly in babyhood when they clung to their mother for dear life. Most of their food came from the trees and they discovered that their hands could be used to gather food as well as cling to branches – and to each other. They became less dependent on all four limbs to maintain balance. They learnt how to squat on their haunches and free both hands for eating. They had few enemies in their tree-top hiding places – the greatest risk was of falling. Their eyes developed stereoscopic vision in order to judge distances more accurately. Brain size increased to cope with processing of all the sensory information needed to jump accurately from branch to branch. Eye-hand co-ordination became extremely important to avoid falling to one's death. Arboreal life laid the foundations for man the tool user.

Primate reproduction

The primates modified the mammalian reproduction system to suit their different needs. The most significant change was the evolution of a unicornate uterus; a female bearing only one child at a time (as nearly all primates do) needed only one womb cavity. (Lower mammals have a Y shaped, two-horned uterus.) There was also a change in the way a foetus lay in the womb. Foetuses of lower mammals tend to curl up in the shape of a cylinder, but primate foetuses curl up into an oval. These two changes opened the way towards an improvement in the working of the uterus at childbirth. The uterus and the foetal position evolved together to fit together more closely, allowing the uterus to play a more directive role in labour.

The uterus is the most complex organ in the body and undergoes enormous changes in pregnancy: it changes its size, shape, type of muscle fibre and its susceptibility to the influence of many different hormones. The biochemistry of the pregnant and labouring uterus is extremely complex and it seems likely that natural selection has favoured giving the womb a more positive role in labour. Rather than simply relieving itself of its contents in what could be a relatively simple manoeuvre, like squeezing toothpaste out of a tube, it seems that primate uterine muscle actively directs and turns the foetus as it expels it. In lower primates with relatively smaller heads than man this may not have been

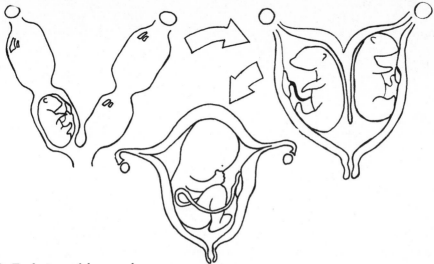

1: Evolution of the womb

a biological necessity, but it opened the door to the safer birth of primates with even larger skulls. Natural selection allowed the mutation to a unicornate uterus because it favoured smaller litter sizes; and fewer infants meant better individual quality of maternal care. The paternal instinct was not yet developed enough to favour twins other than by accident – and besides he could not feed the babies.

The safest way to protect an infant when living in a tree is to carry it around all the time. This close physical contact for prolonged periods of time led to the juxtaposition of touch and maternal behaviour. Infants who learnt better how to cling on to their mother survived; infants letting go fell to their deaths. The close physical relationship between mother and child thus persisted long past life in the womb. It led to a close emotional relationship and we start to see the evolution of human social functioning. Primates still spend much time in close physical contact grooming each other, not just to remove parasites but be-cause it strengthens social ties.

In order to deliver infants with larger brains and consequently larger skulls there were selection pressures to give birth increasingly early in foetal life and to delay more and more physical development until after the birth. This had the disadvantage of making offspring dependant on their mothers for longer, and further decreasing the *quantity* of offspring a mother could raise in her lifetime – a chimpanzee in the wild produces an infant only once every two years. But this disadvantage was outweighed by the *quality* of the infant that was produced. The amount of time that an infant could spend on learning through play was greatly increased. Mature animals fending for themselves must devote much effort to finding food. Primate mothers free their infants from much responsibility for everyday survival giving them time to play and learn; and the delayed onset of sexual maturation frees the young from the distractions of sex.

The selection pressures for maternal behaviour were at least as important as those for producing infants with larger brains; a delinquent mother who left her infants to their fate would leave no offspring. Harlow's famous experiments on the effects of maternal deprivation in Rhesus monkeys showed that monkeys raised without a mother were themselves unable to mother their offspring. Indeed these monkeys lacked even the social skills necessary to conceive offspring of their own, and when they conceived as a result of scientifically engineered "rape" they were unable to mother their infants. These experiments show that, at least in part, primate maternal behaviour is learnt from the mother's own experience of being mothered – an acquired behaviour rather than an innate behaviour. The experience of being mothered appears to be important in the ability to perform the sex act. There is no *biological* pathway for the inheritance of acquired behaviour but there is a *social* pathway for the natural selection of maternal behaviour in primates. Maternal behaviour is also profoundly influenced by hormones which are under genetic control.

The emergence of man – classic view

There is a twelve million year gap in the fossil record which has mystified most palaeontologists for years. The vast tropical forests of the Mesozoic era retreated and the grassy plains of the savannah intruded forcing some primates to leave their tree-top homes and venture out into the wider world. The smaller tropical forests could no longer support all their inhabitants and, life being what it is, the weakest were thrown out and left to their fate. The standard story is that these outcasts took to life on the ground with only their wits for weapons. They became scavengers and ate anything that was to hand in order to survive. The problems of life on the ground were very different from those encountered in arboreal life. Instead of clambering around among the branches, they had to develop a new way of moving, and some chose bipedal walking and thus kept their hands free. The primates had not evolved to run fast to escape from predators, neither to use their teeth as weapons, nor their noses to scent danger or dinner. They compensated for these disadvantages by developing cunning – they learnt to use their hands to throw stones at predators and eventually to make traps and to hunt. They learnt to work in teams to outwit their prey. Those who were cunning survived while the simpletons starved. There was yet another increase in brain power and relative skull size and, most important, the evolution of consciousness, abstract thought, and speech. Once man could talk he had an enormous advantage over the rest of the animal world and gradually, over hundreds of thousands of years *Homo sapiens* emerged and conquered his world. Teamwork was of the utmost importance in this dangerous new world. Males fended off intruders leaving females free to gather food and care for their children.

The emergence of woman – another perspective

The other story of man's evolutionary breakthrough has still not been accepted into the anthropological literature but makes a lot more sense. In *The Descent of Woman*, Elaine Morgan tells the tale of a flight to the seaside and a semi-aquatic existence for twelve million years. This theory was first mooted by Sir Alister Hardy in 1960, a scientist better known now for his interest in the biology of man's soul, which perhaps accounts for the scepticism that greeted his theory. Elaine Morgan took up the fight in 1972 and presented her own compelling account which extended Hardy's theory and used it to account for all manner of physical and psychological peculiarities of the human race, putting women and babies firmly in the anthropological picture. The theory accounts for a naked ape with a full head of hair – useful stuff for grabbing hold of if you are a baby. It does not really matter if daddy is balding. Not being able to feed you, he does not take much notice of you until you can play his rough and tumble games. Upright walking, the streamlined human nose and the weeping and frowning human being are all part of the move towards becoming amphibious. A seaside life was nearly as safe as life in the forest; most predators would not venture near the water so children paddled happily in the shallows while their mothers gathered shellfish, cracking them open with pebbles, learning to use tools. Seafood is said to be highly nutritious for brains.

Perhaps we learnt to love dolphins at this stage in our history – they came and played joyous games with us which we have never forgotten.

There were caves at the seaside for shelter at night. Much as we loved the water, we never became fully aquatic. We emerged, fully fledged human beings, from twelve million years of adaptation towards a watery life but fate played a cruel trick. The ice age dawned and the sea became too cold to swim in so we took our families inland again. Nobody has found fossil clues to this existence, our remains were given a natural sea burial but there seems to be no end of human fossils found in caves.

We might finally have found a clue to pain in childbirth. Seaside woman laboured and gave birth in the water which was the perfect medium for allowing freedom of movement and relieving aches and pains. Perhaps the curse of Eve was the journey back to land, but it did not stop us producing children. We went forth and multiplied.

Human Reproduction

It is often thought that man's increased brain size accounts for the problems of human childbirth but this is not the main cause. Mammalian reproduction seems to have been very efficient at producing offspring with increasingly larger brains. There may have been other mechanisms for producing large brained animals but, if there were, they were not favoured by natural selection. As we have seen in this brief résumé of man's animal roots, natural selection had already found a way of combining reproductive efficiency with increased brain size – prolonged infancy coupled with increased maternal responsibility. It is thought that the genetic mechanism involved in causing an infant to be born at an earlier stage of development was relatively simple. The study of embryonic development shows that the brain is differentiated almost at once and takes up a large proportion of the foetus but that throughout gestation this proportion progressively diminishes.

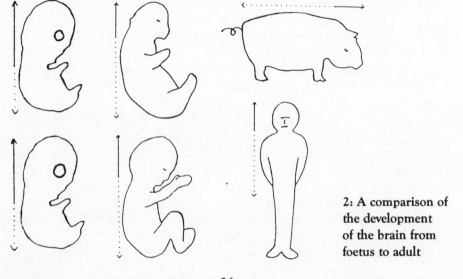

2: A comparison of the development of the brain from foetus to adult

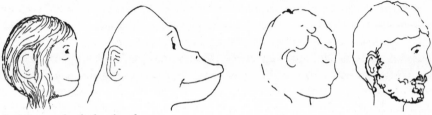

3: Man – the baby faced ape

Man's skull and face resemble skulls and faces of embryos of lower animals. Man is the baby faced ape; he is born at an earlier stage of foetal development; before the bones of his skull have fused together thus allowing the head to mould during labour.

Bipedalism

However, there was a major physical problem to be overcome and that was the physical changes brought about by walking upright. Bipedalism led to a major restructuring of the pelvis and it is from this stage of man's history that the so-called mechanical problems of human childbirth have stemmed. Vertebrates were not designed to walk on their hind legs. The spine in most vertebrates may be imagined as a bridge with the weight of the body firmly supported on four pillars. The animal has a wide base on which to support its weight and the centre of gravity is near ground level. Walking on two legs presents mechanical problems – a smaller base on which to balance and the total body weight now supported on two legs instead of four. The spinal column changed from being a washing line from which to suspend most of the body weight to being a flag pole with the head as the finial.

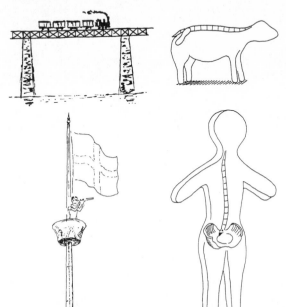

4a: The pillars of a bridge can support the weight of a train, a quadruped's legs support his weight easily

4b: The pelvis is like a crow's nest. It is firmly attached to the spine and supports body weight near to the centre of gravity. It helps man to perform his everyday balancing act of standing upright.

One by-product of the change in the spine is the human tendency towards slipped discs. The human spine gradually evolved to become S shaped to cope with the balancing act required to maintain an upright posture. The evolutionary trends can be seen in the development of a baby's spine. At birth the human spine is arched. At about three months old the first part of the S curve is added at the neck enabling the baby to raise its head and at about one year old the second curve develops in the middle of the back and the baby is ready to stand. The foot evolved from a grasping organ to a weight-bearing platform early in the process of the differentiation of man from ape.

Bipeds had to develop a structure for supporting the weight of the abdominal contents and transferring the weight to the feet. There were enormous changes to the pelvis. It underwent radical changes in a relatively short time. The net result was a 90° rotation backwards and a further change in the spine; the coccyx, the vestigial tail, was tucked out of the way of the birth canal. The pelvis changed from a structure giving kick off power to the hind legs to a basin for supporting the contents of the abdomen – which for women included a baby and it appurtenances. At the same time it had to continue to allow a safe passage for the birth of infants – women need a rounder pelvis for birthing the baby. Evolution solved these conflicting selection pressures with a compromise in women. The male human pelvis is better adapted to running while the female pelvis has continued to provide a larger basin for carrying children and a safe birth canal.

The existence of major sex differences in the human pelvis shows just how important the opposing selection pressures were to facilitate bipedalism on the one hand, and to provide a safe birth canal on the other. Not only has natural selection had time enough to provide for female needs, but also enough time for the male pelvis to adapt better to bipedalism.

The evolution of the female pelvis must have come first since safe birth must be a far more important survival factor than improvement in walking – we are born before we can walk – the survival value of upright walking is not seen until the child is a year old or more. Moreover, mammalian embryos are female by default – the development of a male body depends on the presence of male sex hormones. In the absence of these hormones an embryo will develop a female body, even if it has a male genotype. Male bodies are therefore adaptations to the female body.

If there has been enough evolutionary time for male pelvic structure, with its bias towards faster running, to be differentiated from female pelvic structure, with its bias towards safe birth, we can assume that natural selection has given women the right pelvis for the job of childbearing. Natural selection could only favour those apes mutating towards bipedalism capable of being born alive without killing their mothers in the process. An increasingly erect posture would have been of no use to a stillborn child. Natural selection had to favour safe birth before bipedalism.

(Differentiation of the pelvis continues after birth and male and female sex hormones also have an affect on behaviour. We have no way of knowing the genetically inherited behaviours for urination and defecation in humans, but behavioural scientists know that a male dog deprived of androgen at puberty will continue to squat to urinate as he did as a puppy. It is generally supposed that the change to cocked leg urination resulted from a need to mark territory more accurately; however, I think that the default mechanism for urination is squatting because this widens the pelvic girdle and makes birth easier for females. Once the male dog's body has received enough androgen to be absolutely certain of its masculinity and to know that it will not have to give birth, it can abandon the default squatting position and adopt a urination position of secondary reproductive importance.)

Evolutionary change is slow and many other changes related to enabling the successful emergence of man were taking place at the same time. The chance of this transitional man evolving and becoming well established would have been reduced enormously if most babies were stillborn and many women died in childbirth. I find it impossible to believe that the strength of the forces of natural selection that led to a radically changed pelvis for bipedalism ignored the needs of the child-bearing woman. When seen from the viewpoint of evolution the argument that human females have a genetically ill-adapted pelvis for childbearing just does not hold water. Yet one hears this thesis all too often from obstetricians extolling the virtues of modern scientific childbirth.

Bipedalism causes other problems in man. Since the position of the head and heart have changed radically relative to the ground, man's heart has to work much harder for the brain to be supplied adequately with oxygen; man is more likely to suffer heart disease. The vascular system is relatively ill-adapted, man has a tendency towards varicose veins. These drawbacks may themselves have led to a change in man's personality. Man has been described as possessing a restless personality constantly looking for things to stimulate him and keeping him on the move – thus aiding blood circulation. Indeed, in old age when man is no longer able to maintain an active lifestyle, he becomes more prone to heart disease. Perhaps the restless activity was a biological necessity to maintain optimal blood circulation and increased stimulation of the brain was a by-product. Man's increased restlessness also gave him more learning opportunities. The more he moved around in the world, the more he learned about it.

An upright posture led to changes in the character of the uterine tissue. Women have far more and stronger connective tissue around the opening of the womb, the cervix, than do other mammals. This tissue is needed to keep the foetus inside against the increased force of gravity brought about by postural changes. The human female uterus is qualitatively different from the uteri of lower animals.

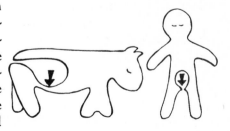

5: New forces on cervix experienced by a biped

Brain size

Homo sapiens is not the only example of a primate with a large brain evolving. Neanderthal man, who survived and reproduced successfully for about 100,000 years had a larger brain (1,650 cc) and was shorter than modern man (around 5 ft tall). Neanderthal man became extinct with the onset of the last glacial period of the Ice Age, possibly he was driven from his European home by *Homo sapiens* himself. Inefficient childbearing is not likely to have been the reason for his extinction. The above argument for the co-evolution of pelvic shape and bipedalism applies equally to the evolution of a larger brain. Apes mutating towards larger brain size had to be born alive before using their increased brain capacity to aid their survival. Natural selection solved this problem partly by folding the brain in concertina fashion. The study of fossil skulls shows an increasingly complex pattern of ridges inside the skull reflecting the increasing complexity of the brain itself. The human brain has a much larger surface area than ape brains but skull size has not increased commensurately with surface area.

The relative size of man's brain seems to have mattered less towards the latter days of man's evolution than the development of specific areas within his brain – yet more specialisation to make individuals better able to adapt to their environment. This final specialisation led to the most significant difference between man and the rest of the animal kingdom. It was the development of the speech areas of the brain: the seat of rationalism. This development was qualitatively different from all that preceded it – once man could communicate effectively he could share in the experience of other individuals. Knowledge pertinent to survival could be pooled. Information could be exchanged regarding resources necessary for survival, for example water or food; and dangerous factors in the environment, for example the presence of predators. Children could be taught by word of mouth instead of by example, and the evolution of culture could start. Man could adapt himself even better to his environment without having to wait for the slow course of natural selection to throw up the odd mutation and reshuffle the existing genetic material.

I suggest that the supposed problems with childbirth are the result of this last adaptation. Childbirth, essentially a physiological process under the control of the subconscious mind, gradually came to be influenced too much by the conscious mind. In the Garden of Eden, Eve ate of the tree of knowledge and learnt to fear childbirth. The true curse of Eve was not that the mechanism of childbirth itself underwent a sudden major change, or even that she had to abandon water birth, but that she discovered her nakedness and became ashamed of her body and its natural functions. As Darwin has said nature does not make jumps. The jump is man-made. Woman discovered the pain that goes hand-in-hand with fear. By treating the pain rather than removing its underlying cause, man's attempts to improve on nature have been doomed to failure. (Although it would be fair to say that man's failure rate is better than it used to be – if only physical outcomes are taken into account.)

Population growth

There are other reasons for supposing that childbirth is not as dangerous as it is made out to be. For populations merely to stand still each woman has to produce at least two children. Replacement level was probably a great deal higher than that – not only do children have to be born alive but they must also live to reach the age of reproduction themselves. Man has a prolonged infancy and a large proportion of his life is spent in childhood. Children are unable to reproduce and have a higher risk of accidental death than adults, having had less time to learn from their mistakes.

Women spend a greater proportion of their lives than men unable to reproduce; men can continue to father children into their nineties but women reach the menopause at around the age of forty-five. By contrast, domestic cats can have their first litter at the age of a year or less and spend the next nine years having kittens – a cat spends less than a tenth of her life on growth to reach reproductive maturity. A human female reaches her reproductive capabilities at about 15 and the menopause at around 45 – she has already spent a third of her life barren and may live for another thirty years. She is fertile for less than half her life and even then has long periods of breastfeeding induced infertility.

I would guess that, for man to maintain a stable population, replacement level would have been at least three children; for him to multiply as he did it must have been nearer half a dozen. Life was cruel and hard before man had fire to warm him and tools to help him hunt his food more effectively. The first man did not have the benefit of modern obstetrics and yet he managed to be fruitful and multiply. In fact his wife sometimes presented him with *too many* children – there is evidence of infanticide in early civilisations as well as in some present day cultures, including our own according to the anti-abortion lobby.

Peculiarities of human reproduction

Mating position

Nearly all other animals mate with the male entering the female from behind, but most humans prefer the face-to-face position. In the missionary position men and women can *talk to each other* while making love. Sexual intercourse in humans creates and strengthens social bonds between man and woman, and social bonds are forged in language. The social bonds are all important in ensuring that women are not left alone to bring up their children. Families need fathers, and face-to-face mating helps to turn a biological father into a social father.

Feeding position

Likewise our breasts are so placed that we can feed our babies while maintaining eye contact and can communicate with our offspring in between bouts of sucking. Feeding is the first event in our social calendar.

Fertility control

Most other female primates ovulate within a few days, or at most, weeks after giving birth but in humans lactation inhibits ovulation for between six months and three years, depending on the amount of suckling, which allows the mother to concentrate her physical and mental resources on the existing baby before embarking on another. This is another example of selection pressures towards producing higher quality children rather than more children.

The natural selection of grandmothers

As I have pointed out in the preceding section, human females spend a large proportion of their lives unable to produce children. Why can women live so long after their child-bearing days are over? One might think that natural selection would have no mechanism for ensuring the survival of post-menopausal women; older women use up valuable environmental resources that could perhaps be better spent on feeding children and people still able to reproduce. However, grandmothers are notoriously fond of their grandchildren, who contain about a quarter of their genes. There is a selective advantage for children who have grandmothers still alive. Grandmothers represent an extra pair of hands for the mother. A mother who is less worn out by her maternal responsibilities will survive longer to produce more children and pass on more of her own mother's genes. Grandmothers also provide their grandchildren with that most valuable resource - time to play. Grandmothers were the first teachers, the first play group leaders and the first nannies; they are grossly undervalued in modern society. The modern cult of youth is another retrograde step for mankind. Grandmothers embody an enormous fount of wisdom, largely untapped now that each generation has its own childcare guru. Dr Spock, Hugh Jolly and Penelope Leach have displaced granny. No wonder she feels an outcast.

Loss of seasonal breeding patterns

There is no biological reason why humans should indulge in sex at all times in the menstrual cycle even when there is no chance of the woman becoming pregnant. Humans also indulge when the woman is already pregnant (so also do rats - but the male rat thereby causes the female to abort unless the offspring she is carrying belong to him). The evolutionary explanation is that intercourse strengthens the social ties between man and woman. Orgasm in both men and woman leads to the production of pleasure hormones. Shared pleasure leads to stronger bonds. Human females need their partners for long periods of time to support them while they care for their children.

On a more mundane note, frequent intercourse will greatly reduce the probability that a man will be cuckolded. Primitive man's genes needed to know that his wife would be faithful or he might waste his time feeding some other man's children. The development of paternal behaviour was crucial to the evolution of a species where both mother and children were dependent on male protection for years at a time. Fathers also had more time for rough and tumble play - another social activity.

Dowdy males instead of dowdy females

It has often been pointed out that the human species is one of only a few species where the male is considered less intrinsically attractive than the female. Women's bodies have been worshipped as epitomising beauty and fertility since man began to draw and sculpt. But the body must be firm and youthful, capable of mating, childbirth and suckling. Men gain the upper hand with distinguished good looks in middle age when modern woman is tempted by plastic surgery and rejuvenating face creams.

Women have a vested interest in keeping their partners to support them and their children and must therefore take pains to continue to be sexually attractive and to pleasure their husband in case he decides to go off and father more children with a younger woman who can provide him with yet more children. A woman who continues to be sexually attractive when her child-bearing years are nearly over is able to raise more children than one who does not bother. Woman's good looks tend to last only as long as she is able to bear children whereas men tend to stay sexually attractive for longer. Nature will help women only as long as they can bear children – there is a strong genetic pressure for a man to desert his wife for a younger woman. (I will refrain from further comment.)

Differences in sexual needs

The male sexual urge seems to be more immediate than the female sexual urge for humans. Many males may be relieved by "wham, bam, thank you ma'm" attitude to sex but most females need a more gentle approach to love making, with more foreplay to prepare their bodies for the sexual act itself. This is one area where human differ most from animals and it can be accounted for by the increased human female need for long-term protection for herself and her young. It gives human females a chance to choose their mate more carefully with regard to their long-term needs. If a male is prepared to give her what she wants in intercourse, then perhaps he will consider her wider needs as well as his own in the future. Also prolonged lovemaking strengthens emotional ties between man and woman which will be useful when a child is born to them and the woman needs emotional and material support in caring for her young.

Genetic Accidents

You might well be forgiven for thinking that I have so fallen in love with natural selection as the mechanism for producing healthy children that I am blind to its faults, so I had better put the record straight. Of course genetic accidents occur. Natural selection depends on them. Recessive lethal genes are the price we have to pay for maintaining genetic variability. Over evolutionary time overall mutation rates have fallen as the earth has acquired a protective layer of ozone which screens out harmful radiation from the sun which increases mutations. Man is in grave danger of increasing the mutation rate through profligate use of fossil fuels and CFCs which destroy the ozone layer. He is also increasing genetic risks to his children by injudicious use of medical X-rays, most of which are unnecessary, and by continuing to develop nuclear arms and nuclear power. For individuals, genetic accidents are life shattering but, as my fictitious obstetrician said in the previous chapter, nature does not care about the individual. Neither, might I add, does the present in-stitutionalised cattle market attitude of modern obstetricians towards childbirth.

43

There are three basic types of genetic accident: the coming together of two recessive detrimental genes in a foetus, for example Tay Sach's disease; the mutation of a previously normal gene into a bad gene, for example some kinds of dwarfism; and chromosomal mistakes taking place when the sperm and egg unite, for example Down's syndrome.

Terminology is misleading. People usually take "congenital" to mean genetically inherited but congenital merely means present at birth. And disabilities present at birth may have genetic or environmental causes. Some congenital abnormalities are caused by lack of an essential nutrient at a certain stage in the development of the foetus. These represent faults with the environment of the womb itself. For example neural tube defects, including spina bifida, are thought to result from a lack of folic acid in the mother's diet in the first few weeks of pregnancy. There appear to be few genetic accidents regarding childbirth itself. It used to be fashionable to blame problems in childbirth on a genetically small pelvis, but it is now known that nearly all women produce babies to fit their pelvis. Severely deformed pelves are caused by poor nutrition in childhood rather than genetic mistakes – an environmental problem rather than a genetic one. Other congenital abnormalities may even be caused by birth itself. If the baby is deprived of oxygen for too long at some time in labour then part of his brain may die, labour itself is another environmental hazard to overcome. Some congenital disabilities may be caused by doctors themselves. No one knows quite what the physical effects of forceps and caesarean deliveries are and some of the ill effects may be labelled congenital, falsely implying a genetic origin for some birth accidents. For example, a baby may be born with respiratory distress syndrome (RDS), poor lung function. This is congenital in that it is present at birth but may be directly caused by inducing premature labour. In the 1970s the incidence of RDS escalated but today no one suggests that the prime cause of this rise was genetic; on the contrary, it is agreed that it was caused by over zealous induction programmes.

The Rhesus Factor

The genetic control of the Rhesus factor in blood is one of the few examples of the failure of natural selection to ensure safe childbirth for the child. It is often given as an example of man's superiority over nature and the prevention of Rhesus disease is indeed one of the real triumphs of modern obstetrics. However, natural selection only has to do well enough to account for the continuing existence of the detrimental gene and there are many ways in which natural selection has avoided wiping out the Rh-negative gene. First, barring accidents in the womb, the first child escapes the ill effects of the gene since the most likely time for Rhesus sensitisation of the mother to occur is at childbirth, a situation that has not yet been encountered in a first pregnancy. Second, some Rh-negative women will mate with Rh-negative men so their children will escape altogether. Third, the woman's mate may be heterozygous for the Rhesus factor in which case there is a 50% chance for each pregnancy that the resulting child would be Rh-negative. Finally, if a Rh-positive child's blood is of a different blood group the mother's blood will recognise the foetal blood as foreign and destroy it before there is a chance to form antibodies against the Rh-negative component of the foetal blood. Today only 15% of Rh-negative mothers producing Rh-positive offspring would become sensitised even without treatment although 75% of their children are likely to be phenotypically Rh-positive.

There may well be a beneficial effect of the Rh-negative gene that also helped its survival in the gene pool in the same way that there is with the gene for sickle cell anaemia, which protects against malaria. There are many ways that the Rh-negative gene could have slipped through the net of natural selection.

Its existence shows quite categorically that nature does not know best for the individual. Nature does not mind that 1 in 200 pregnancies are likely to result in an infant with haemolytic disease – the gene is lethal for only a small proportion of progeny. It could well be that natural selection has already played a part in reducing the incidence of Rhesus iso-immunisation in pregnancy. In other parts of the world, populations contain far fewer people with Rh-negative blood groups.

There are other rare blood incompatibility disorders of pregnancy; rare enough for nature to ignore the consequences for individuals. Another genetic anomaly is the increased risk of thrombosis following delivery. This is a by-product of bipedalism – nature ensures that the risk of post-partum haemorrhage is reduced by raising clotting factors in the blood in the last month of pregnancy and for six weeks postnatally but in humans the heart is a long way away from the feet and has to work very hard to maintain circulation; man has an innate tendency to thrombosis.

Conclusion

It seems that the emergence of an intelligent being able to use his hands for tool-making, his brain for problem solving, his tongue for talking and his heart for loving was the result of a series of happy accidents. In short these were adding instinctive behaviour to the behavioural repertoire of reflex actions; the choice of a method of reproduction that allowed an increase in brain size; and even the evolution of a creature that needed to be on the move constantly to keep his brain supplied with oxygen. All these factors gave man the chance to develop his intellectual powers to the full. At each step on the genetic road towards man there were choices to be made. Sometimes the benefits of a particular option were not seen for thousands of generations; the mutation was selected for other immediate reasons, but the seeds of man's biology were laid. Perhaps some dormant genes were switched on again; mutations had unforeseen advantages that came into their own millions of years later.

Looking at man's biological heritage with the benefit of hindsight one can be forgiven for thinking that Nature had a grand purpose; that man is the culmination of the powers of evolution. I must admit that a large part of me wants to believe in the hand of God directing the course of evolution to create a creature worthy of Himself, but the scientific evidence is against this. Nature's accidents are themselves evidence of the blind forces of natural selection – proof of our biological heritage.

However, the mechanism of human childbirth is not one of Nature's accidents. Natural childbirth has evolved to suit the species and if mankind chooses to ignore her advice and interfere with her workings we must not complain about the consequences. We have only ourselves to blame.

2   Instinct and Stress

There once was a man who said, "Damn!
It is borne in upon me that I am
An engine that moves
In predestinate grooves,
I'm not even a bus I'm a tram."

M.E.Hare (1886-1967)

Both my mother and myself were given dire warnings of what could go wrong with childbirth by our medical advisors, and we both found reassurance in seeing how easily our domestic pets reproduced – in my mother's case guinea pigs, and in my own our cat, who produced her first family a month before my first child was born. Neither the guinea pig nor the cat had the help of a doctor nor even a midwife and neither could have known what was in store for them, yet they managed all the same. We had seen the cat looking for a safe place for her kittens and had provided her with a kitten box in the weeks preceding the birth. When her time came, and the first kitten popped out in the middle of our bedroom floor, she looked rather surprised but picked the kitten up by the scruff of its neck and carried it to her kitten box where she delivered the next one. There was no agonised mewling, quite the contrary – the purring had to be heard to be believed, and she was so proud of herself. If animals know instinctively how to give birth and care for their young, why do humans not know? Or do they?

What is instinct?
Instinctive behaviour is behaviour motivated not by conscious rational thought, but by subconscious direction from the brain. Most of the time we are unaware of this internal motivation but, occasionally, instinctive cues cross the threshold into consciousness and we are aware of "feeling compelled" to act in a particular way. All behaviour has some kind of motivation. The brain provides nervous and hormonal motivation such as hunger and thirst, pain-avoidance, the sexual urge, the fight or flight response to danger and so on. Most of the time our behaviour is determined by rational, social and cultural factors but these factors can still be overruled when the brain deems it necessary. When our biological instinctive behaviour gains the upper hand and we are given instinctive behavioural instructions, the brain also prepares our body for the necessary action. If we need to act fast to escape from danger, our skeletal muscles are given increased glucose for energy. The brain is constantly trying to make us act to match our external environment to our internal bodily needs. When the state of imbalance has been corrected the brain regains its equilibrium, the nervous or hormonal motivation is taken away and the compulsive feeling disappears.

The brain is the body's on-board computer, constantly receiving signals from the rest of the body concerning both the internal state of the body and the external environment, processing the information and sending out signals to enable the body to adapt.

Instinctive motherhood

In the fight for survival and in the quest for reproduction, behaviour was of paramount importance and the force of natural selection was as powerful for the selection of appropriate behaviour as it was for efficient bodily function. This is as true for maternal behaviour as it is for the sexual urge. No matter how spacious the pelvis and how well developed the uterine muscles, the safe delivery of an infant depends as much on behaviour during pregnancy and childbirth as on the physical design of the reproductive organs. Efficient bodily function depends on appropriate behaviour. Survival of the offspring to adulthood also depends on appropriate behaviour of the mother. Offspring of mothers who lacked the maternal instinct would die. In nature, mothering must be an instinctive process rather than under the control of consciousness. Before man could talk and exchange knowledge his women could deliver their babies and bring them up. It seems unlikely that in the relatively short period of time between the Garden of Eden and the present day the genes for instinctive mothering should have been lost.

Genes and behaviour

How can our genes determine our behaviour? Indeed, is it true that man's genes still determine his behaviour or has he risen above behaving on a purely instinctive level? We have not been emancipated from our instincts but rational behaviour chosen through free will has been laid on top of a complex, genetically determined behavioural system.

Being rational human beings, we do not like to think of our behaviour as being under the control of animal instincts and yet it is obvious, to the advertising industry if to no one else, that much of our behaviour is at least influenced, if not controlled, by our subconscious mind. Advertisers sell us products by stimulating instincts for hunger, thirst, sex, pursuit of pleasure and security. We like to think that we have risen above behaving at a purely instinctive level – and so we have to some extent – we can modify our behaviour in all sorts of ways: contact lens users can overcome the innate reflex of the eye to an approaching foreign body; and we can train ourselves to overcome instinctive fears, for example fear of flying, through behaviour therapy. However, if we think that we have outgrown our instincts we delude ourselves.

Behavioural conditioning

There is a strong genetic influence on social behaviour. Man evolved as a social animal, an animal who was responsive to peer pressure, who was happy when he pleased his companions and psychologically stressed when excluded by them. We have a biological need for the companionship and approval of others and we start to learn this at our mother's breast. If we make her angry she may refuse to feed us, indeed stress hormones caused by her anger will inhibit the flow of milk and she may be physically unable to lactate.

Most of our social training is behavioural conditioning – learning to inhibit selfish instinctive responses. In man's early days this behavioural conditioning was accomplished in the home and immediate community but, as man became civilised, the complex institutions of the church, the state, law and education evolved for mass behavioural conditioning. Many people still feel instinctively that the home and local community have a greater effect on behaviour than institutional conditioning, formal education and the law of the land. Nearly everyone acknowledges the importance of home background in creating good citizens. Community policing is seen as more effective than policing at a distance. Behavioural conditioning operates through rewarding good behaviour and punishing bad behaviour and if those rewards and punishments are meted out by parents and acquaintances they will have a stronger effect on behaviour than more formal sanctions. Peer pressure is stronger than the force of the law.

Part of man's very success in populating the earth is owed to individuals learning how to behave altruistically for the benefit of society – pooling resources and sharing knowledge. But when the individual can no longer see the connection between his own community and the larger community of the state then the sanctions of the state become less effective and there is a tendency to lawlessness.

The psychological need for approval by our peers is the biological foundation of altruism. We become distressed when reprimanded and thrive on approval.

Physiology of behaviour

Survival and reproduction depend not only on a healthy body but on appropriate behaviour. Behaviour can be innate, instinctive and learned. We inherit a brain and nervous system that is already wired up to produce some innate behaviour and which has an enormous capacity for making new connections to encode learned behaviour in memory so that we may learn from experience. Our bodies are richly supplied with nerves to send and receive information enhancing our chances of survival and reproduction. We are born with a biochemical hormone system, the endocrine system, and all hormones have a great deal of influence on our behaviour.

At puberty, the endocrine system is enhanced by an increase in the production of the sex hormones which evolved to maximise our reproductive potential by influencing behaviour likely to lead to the birth of children.

Our genes encode instructions for appropriate behaviour by dictating the anatomy of the nervous system and providing templates for the production of specific biochemicals: neurotransmitters, which make chemical links between nerve cells; and hormones which use blood to pass messages. Our bodies appear to work in much the same way as animals' bodies, or medical scientists would not spend so much time doing experiments on animals. Hormones affect both body and mind in animals and there is no reason why the behavioural effects of hormones observed in animals should not manifest themselves in human beings. Women suffering from pre-menstrual tension or going through the menopause are only too aware of the behavioural effects of sex hormones such as oestrogen and progesterone. But effects of hormones upon behaviour are not confined to women or indeed to sex hormones. Our brains and bodies are bathed in hormones from birth to the grave and they influence our body, our personality and our behaviour in the most unexpected ways throughout our lives.

Nearly all textbooks on hormones and behaviour give most space to animal behaviour with a short paragraph at the end of each section about human behaviour. Scientists are extremely reluctant to talk about hormones and human behaviour; indeed some of them go so far as to state that human behaviour is definitely not controlled by hormones but by learning. This is particularly so in the case of reproduction and mothering: "Certainly, the behaviour of human parents is not controlled by innate factors... Learning seems to be more important than hormonal activation." writes one male behavioural physiologist (Carlson, 1991). This attitude appears rather dated in the light of the links between learning and stress hormones. As a mother I find it almost unbelievable that anyone could think that human maternal behaviour is *not* affected by hormones. Even doctors recognise the hormonal motivation of the nesting instinct and some studies report disturbed human maternal instincts following caesarean section instead of delivery by the vaginal route which stimulates mothering hormones in animals. The widespread effects of hormones on maternal behaviour in animals, both before and after birth, have been well researched. However, the sweeping assumption that hormones do not affect human maternal behaviour has no grounding in observed fact and is a politically inspired statement to defend current obstetric practice and to appease some feminists.

In the vast literature on the endocrinology of reproductive behaviour there is precisely nothing on hormones influencing behaviour during birth itself, even for animals. This is an almost unbelievable omission which perhaps reflects the male domination of science. For the behavioural scientists maternal behaviour starts during pregnancy, stops for labour, and continues after the actual birth. For the medical establishment the hormones of pregnancy, childbirth and milk production have only physiological effects – psychological effects are completely ignored, yet a deeper look at birthing hormones in women could help to solve such psychiatric and social problems as postnatal depression, battered babies and the failure-to-thrive syndrome. (Children failing to thrive fall behind set developmental norms for no apparent medical reason.)

Research methodology of hormones and behaviour

Of course it is far easier to do experiments on animals than on humans. Scientists can remove hormone secreting glands, inject hormones into the blood stream or into different parts of the brain. They can manipulate the animal's environment: deprive it of food or drink, change the light/dark cycle, add or remove cage mates and induce stress in various ways – give electric shocks, put a novel stimulus in the cage, or introduce a predator. All these procedures are designed to inflict psychological stress on animals. Some surgical techniques for studying hormone secretion I find hard to stomach. It is difficult to see why these experiments should be done at all if the results are not then used to alleviate human suffering but merely to extend knowledge of pure science. On the other hand, much of the scientific argument in this book derives from such research so I am unable to condemn it outright. I am however appalled that scientists are content to experiment on primates captured in the wild, many of which die before even reaching the scientists' laboratories.

It is not ethical to manipulate the bodies and lives of people, particularly during pregnancy, and thus it is not so easy to see clear cut "cause and effect" relationships of hormones and behaviour in humans. (Cause and effect itself is out of fashion with the scientists these days which accounts for the inverted commas but, like most people, I tend to think in terms of cause and effect. Scientific language, phrases such as "A influences B" are too woolly and can lead to confusion, for example does an increase in A lead to an increase in B or a decrease in B?)

Physiologists can judge the behavioural effects of human hormones by observing people whose hormones are disturbed by disease or surgery, and psychologists can observe people and measure hormone secretion in naturally occurring situations. I feel that there is enough of this psycho-physiological evidence for us to be reasonably sure that the physiological mechanism of instinctive human behaviour is broadly similar to animal instinctive behaviour and that rational behaviour is indeed laid on top of an existing system, and does not supersede it, as is so often assumed. Katherina Dalton has made the largest contribution to hormonal influences on women's behaviour with her work on progesterone and pre-menstrual tension (Dalton, 1984). There is also evidence of the behavioural effects of oestrogen from the literature on the menopause and hormone replacement therapy (Cooper, 1979). But there are some very large gaps in knowledge – the biggest gap of all concerning birth itself.

Despite the lack of hard scientific data, the anecdotal evidence that hormones affect human behaviour in broadly similar ways to their effects on animal behaviour is certainly very strong, particularly for mothering hormones during pregnancy and after birth.

My own method has been to look at the biology of hormone secretion in the same way as do endocrinologists, to look at behaviour as seen by mothers, midwives and psychologists and to try to marry the two together to discover cause and effect relationships between hormone secretion and behaviour. For example one can make an educated guess about the likely hormonal states of mothers following caesarean section with or without trial of labour and relate this to actual observations of behaviour. I have thus made a start on studying the psycho-physiology of human pregnancy, labour and mothering. I emphasize that it is only a start. There are endless possibilities for further research which I hope will be done by anyone who is interested.

Physiology of Instinct

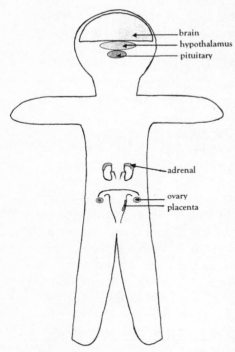

brain
hypothalamus
pituitary

adrenal

ovary
placenta

6: Hormone glands

There are two main physiological systems for receiving and sending the information needed by the brain for it to assess survival needs and prescribe appropriate behaviour. The first is the nervous system; if we touch somehing hot we react almost instantaneously by removing the body part concerned from the source of heat. The second system is the hormone system. This system is slower to react but is capable of a far greater degree of control over our behaviour.

The body's communication networks

Peter Nathan in *The Oxford Companion to the Mind* has compared nerves to telegraph wires and hormones to radio waves. Nerve cells physically connect different parts of the body just as telegraph wires physically connect places on the telephone network. Electrical messages are passed along both. The brain may be thought of as the STD (direct dialling) system. For long-distance calls, which connect places geographically far apart, the connection must be made at a central place, but for local calls one needs only to dial a few numbers and the connection will be made at a local exchange. This is true of nerves also. Some nerves are connected only through the brain whereas others connect locally. The spinal cord acts as a local exchange as well as being a channel to access the brain.

The endocrine, or hormone system, uses the blood circulation system to send and receive its messages. Hormones circulate in the blood and are suffused throughout the body much as radio waves permeate the air. Whether or not a radio wave is translated into sound at a particular place depends on whether there is a radio receiver there; whether it can pick up particular types of transmissions (long, medium, short-wave frequencies or VHF); whether it is switched on; the strength of the signal; and the presence or absence of radio interference.

Hormones also work in this way. Particular hormones, like particular transmission signals, need particular receptors. Some hormones have receptors in many places throughout the body while others have receptors in limited areas. Like radio waves, hormones can suffer from interference with two hormones competing for the same receptor site – one hormone can "jam" another. Some hormones carry instructions to build more receptors for themselves or other hormones at a particular site.

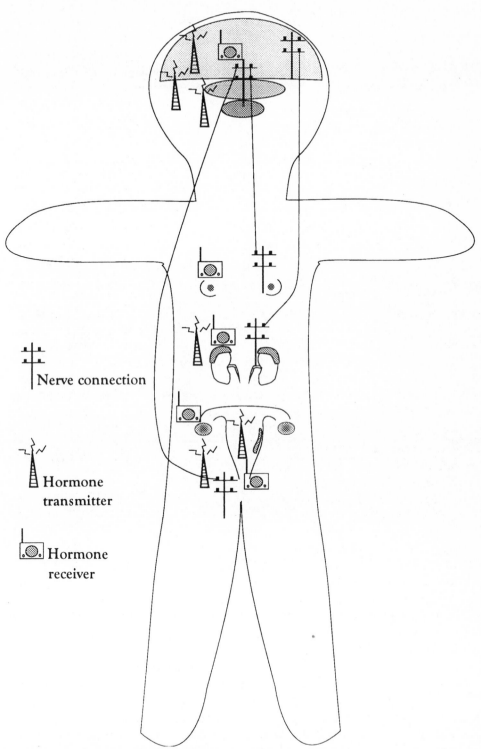

Nerve connection

Hormone
transmitter

Hormone
receiver

7: Nerves physically connect different parts of the body. Hormones enter the
blood system and go all over the body

53

The endocrine system is supervised by the brain itself. The brain is both a transmitter and receiver of hormonal signals. The hypothalamus and pituitary gland are amplification and relay stations for hormones. The brain delegates much responsibility for every day life to automatic controls and interferes only when necessary to preserve life in face of danger.

The nervous system

The nervous system depends on physical connections between nerve cells. If nerve cells touch each other they can pass messages, if they do not touch they cannot. Nerve messages are simple: the nervous system is like a computer in that it depends on physical connections between nerve cells. Likewise, a computer is a complicated series of electrical connections, electrical circuits. Switches that can be on or off. This is a binary code in mathematical terms. Nerve cells are either firing, or they are not. The rate of firing can vary but not the physical effect. The nervous system operates automatically. It screens incoming nerve signals and passes information on to the brain only when firing rates exceed certain thresholds.

Although the human body is far better designed than a computer and contains an enormous number of electrical connections, there is still a limit to the physical capacity of the body and brain as an information processor if only nervous signals are taken into account. The nervous system is too simple to account for the complex behaviour of the bodies and minds of mammals.

The nervous system works quickly and is responsible for fleeting changes in emotional states. There are a limited number of emotional responses to situations – fear, anger, disgust, sadness, surprise and amusement have been suggested by one researcher (Levenson, 1988). Specific facial expressions reflect these emotions and some can be observed universally among mammals, for example bared teeth, while some seem to be specific to primates. Humans are the only primates to frown and weep. Fleeting emotions, being near instantaneous responses to situations, depend on the fast action of the nervous system. The intensity of emotions experienced will depend on the underlying state of arousal of the brain. The stronger the level of arousal, the stronger the response. These quick responses seem to be innate but they last only a few seconds. The next behavioural move will be determined by the brain's interpretation of the emotional situation and its environmental context. The brain considers the emotion in its context, relates these to past experience and decides upon appropriate action. This action is mediated by the hormone system.

The hormone system

Hormones are sent to remote parts of the body in the bloodstream. Whether or not a particular part of the body makes any use of a particular hormonal message carried in the blood depends on whether it has appropriate receptors or receiving stations for that particular hormone in its cells. Cells in different parts of the body react differently to the same hormone. Hormones can carry lots of different messages at the same time and the particular message acted on

54

depends on the particular cell the hormone finds itself in. For example, oestrogen prepares the uterine lining to receive a fertilised egg, prepares uterine muscle for labour contractions, tells bone cells to take up calcium from the blood and switches on manufacture of vaginal lubricants. If enough oestrogen reaches receptors in the brain, libido is increased. Some studies have found that women tend to be more interested in sex around the time of ovulation and just before their period, both situations of high oestrogen. Oestrogen thus has physiological effects in the body and provides psychological motivation in the brain. The increase in sex drive is less marked in women than in animals (Elaine Morgan expounds the reasons in *The Descent of Woman).* Indeed, as with the mothering instinct, it has been said that social factors account for all human motivation for sex. However, social behaviour is itself motivated by hormones.

Bodily functions are controlled by hormones subconsciously and automatically. Only rarely are we aware of the constant automatic work of the hormones which keep the heart and lungs pumping, the gut digesting and a myriad other life-sustaining activities. These hormones are usually secreted automatically on directions from the hypothalamus and the pituitary gland, which control hormone levels, usually without much interference from the on-board computer of the brain.

The hierarchy of organisation of the hormone system is like that of a factory. The endocrine glands are the hired hands who do as they are told, the pituitary gland contains the foremen who oversee production of different sections of the factory according to a given rule book, the hypothalamus is the site manager co-ordinating activity of the factory as a whole, and the brain is the chief executive who makes overall production decisions according to environmental factors such as finance available and market requirements for the product. If money is scarce, production must be geared to make best use of limited resources. When the market is stable there is no need to change overall production but, in an unstable market, the overall manager will need to give constant instructions to the site manager regarding production requirements.

The brain overrules the hypothalamus in the body when environmental conditions are unstable, when the animal is stressed. The brain matches the body's behaviour to the prevailing conditions in the outside world.

The brain is the interface between the nervous system and the endocrine system, both nervous and hormonal information reach the brain. The brain analyses the information it receives from the body itself and from the environment. It transmits nervous and hormonal messages to change behaviour of body and mind to adapt to aid survival.

The brain, therefore, reserves the right to interfere with automatic hormone regulation and can overrule hormone release decisions taken by the hypothalamus and pituitary gland. A healthy body or internal environment is important for survival and reproduction, but so also is the need to escape risks of death that come from outside the body – from the animal's external environment. The brain decides whether to focus energy on the internal environment, processes of *growth, repair and reproduction,* which can be seen as long-term survival strategies; or whether to switch attention to the external environment to deal with dangers, which can be seen as a *short-term survival strategy.*

Stress Hormones and Behaviour

I have no doubt that the mere mention of the word stress sets off a loud groan in many readers. However, stress is "The Disease of Civilisation" according to Dr Michel Odent, and it seems abundantly clear that he is right. I must admit that I too am getting sick and tired of hearing how we must reduce our stress levels to prevent ill health. Mothers of young children in particular feel despair, helplessness and hopelessness at the mere mention of stress itself. Juggling the demands of husband, children and paid employment is enough to drive anyone to distraction. Society makes enormous demands on modern women and gives them scant reward for their pains. They feel guilty if they go out to work, guilty if they stay at home to look after their children, angry at the seemingly endless demands of children and ageing relatives and yet guiltier still if they transfer responsibilities to others. Now they are made to feel guilty about their own increased stress levels which result largely from their care for others. No wonder women are angry!

It may seem a little odd to have an account of stress hormones in a birth book but stress hormones are inextricably linked with reproduction hormones. ß-endorphin, a stress hormone, regulates oestrogen and oxytocin, female reproductive hormones. Prolactin, the main mothering hormone is switched on by the act of becoming a mother and suckling a baby – it is also switched on by stress hormones. The forces of natural selection designed mothers to feel rewarded if they did their job well and to feel psychological stress if they did not. If we understand stress hormones, how they work, and when they are secreted, we can start to make sense of the hormonal mechanisms underlying the behaviour of both the mother and her baby and learn about the effect of stress on their relationship. *We can also begin to understand how the stresses of civilisation and modern maternity practices can interfere with the engineering of childbirth.*

The survival value of stress hormones
I think that we can understand stress hormones and their actions most easily when we ask ourselves why they have evolved at all. Stress hormones have been linked with heart disease, cancer and a multitude of other disorders of civilised man. However, while decreasing the chance of survival in the long term, they greatly enhance short-term survival. In order to be fruitful and multiply animals had not only to reproduce but also to avoid sudden death. They had to develop some mechanism for ensuring short-term survival while continuing to pursue the long-term goal of reproduction.

I think that, generally speaking, we can put behaviour into two categories: short-term survival behaviour and long-term survival behaviour. Animals ignoring their instincts and paying too little attention to short-term survival would risk death; their genes would not be passed on and would disappear from the gene pool. Stress hormones and instincts evolved to enable the animal to make the best possible adaptation to his immediate surroundings in potentially dangerous situations.

Long-term survival

Long-term survival depends on *growth* to reproductive maturity; renewal and *repair* of the body; and *reproduction* to ensure that genes are carried forwards to the next generation. All these functions require food (a source of energy) and other prerequisites for life. Behaviour connected with long-term survival includes searching for sustenance, eating when hungry, digesting food, sleeping when tired and for the female, nurturing the foetus, giving birth, making milk and caring for the young.

Short-term survival

Short-term survival depends on reacting quickly to changes in the environment – forgetting about long-term survival when faced with danger, abandoning growth, repair and reproduction behaviour and putting all available energy into immediate survival. The brain concentrates on short-term survival needs until the danger has passed and, only when it is safe again, does long-term survival behaviour return. Stress hormones switch priorities between immediate survival strategies and long-term growth, repair and reproduction strategies. Loss of appetite, sleeplessness and lack of sex drive are classic symptoms of stress.

Survival priorities and the brain

We saw in the last chapter that mammals were so good at short-term survival, at escaping danger in the environment, that they could afford to produce fewer offspring and yet still prosper. They were better at looking after themselves and better at looking after their offspring, despite an enormous investment in body and time on the part of the mother.

They were better both at observing danger in their surroundings and at acting fast enough to avoid death. They were also capable of learning from their mistakes so that they became able to predict danger (for example, they were able to learn to see, smell or hear a predator before he came too close for comfort) and act before it was too late. All these activities require observing the environment, assessing it for danger, making predictions about the safest strategies, deciding priorities for long-term survival or short-term survival and acting on the net result. This is *information processing* and will be familiar to people working with computers. The larger the computer, the more information it can process. The brain is the body's on-board computer, constantly receiving signals from the body concerning its internal state and signals from the outside world, processing the information and sending out instructions enabling the body to adapt. The stress hormone system is the means by which the brain instructs the body to switch survival strategies.

Stress Hormones

Sudden stress hormones

Adrenaline and noradrenaline are fast acting and can be understood better as an adjunct to the nervous system rather than as true hormones. Noradrenaline is itself also a neurotransmitter, that is, a substance involved in making nerve cells fire. Sudden stress, physical or psychological, leads to a quick secretion of adrenaline and noradrenaline into the blood stream. Nerve cells based in the brain fire a nervous signal directly to the adrenal gland and secretion of adrenaline and noradrenaline is the near instantaneous response. Adrenaline and noradrenaline act on nerve endings throughout the body. They make chemical connections between the nerve endings and cell membranes thus allowing nervous information to reach the cell. Thus, although they are hormones in that they use the blood for transportation, they are released by a nervous message and their effects are predominantly nervous. This is why they act so quickly.

The action of adrenaline and noradrenaline on the muscles of the face is responsible for the facial expressions reflecting the various innate emotional responses.

We are all aware of the consequences of a sudden rush of adrenaline: the heart pounds, we become instantly alert, we may blush as blood rushes to the brain to prepare it for hard work. Adrenaline and noradrenaline have opposite effects on different parts of the body, for example they make the smooth muscle of the heart work harder but stop the smooth muscle of the womb contracting. Adrenaline and noradrenaline affect different body parts differently according to receiving stations for the hormones in a particular place. In some parts, for example the heart, nerve firing will be excitatory and make a body part work harder, but in other parts increased nerve firing is inhibitory and will prevent a body part working. Different parts of the body have evolved differently in their response to adrenaline and noradrenaline in the blood. Adrenaline and noradrenaline elicit reflex behaviours. The sudden stress hormones also have a true hormonal effect of sending a chemical message to the brain telling it to increase production of arousal hormones which will lead to instinctive behaviour.

Arousal hormones

Most people know very little about arousal hormones: the stress hormones with the most pronounced learned instinctive as opposed to reflex behavioural effects. Their actions on both the body and the mind are outlined below.

ACT Hormone

ACT hormone (adrenocorticotropic hormone, more usually known as ACTH) prepares the body and the mind for ACTION. ACT hormone has a message for the mind and a message for the body. The message to the mind is *"arouse yourself, act now to relieve your stress."* ACT hormone prepares the mind for work. It makes us more alert to changes in the environment perceived through the five senses, it switches on instinctive danger-avoiding behaviour and it enhances our memory mechanisms.

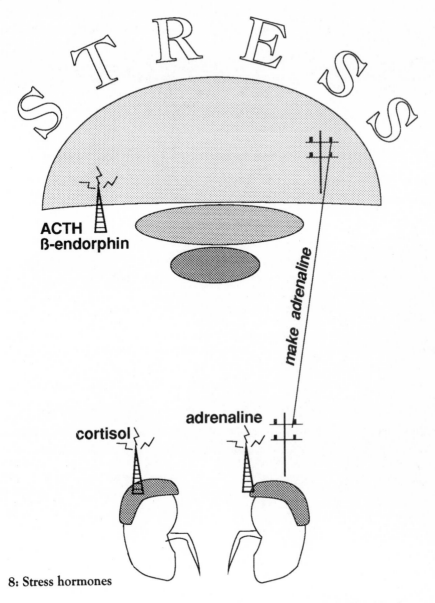

8: Stress hormones

Stress hormones are secreted when the brain thinks that we should take action to avoid danger or to reduce psychological stress. In psychological terms, the less we know about our immediate environment, the more dangerous it may be. The stranger the environment, the more stress hormones are secreted. Stress hormones increase our ability to adapt to new situations and to encode experience in memory so that, when next encountered, the situation will no longer be new and will cause less stress. Learning involves building up a mental picture of the world and how to exist in it. ACT hormone signals that a new situation has arisen. The first priority is to survive the danger but it is also important to remember what we did to cope so that we can use the same strategy next time the situation arises. If we treated every situation as a new situation we would never have the time or energy for growth, repair and reproduction.

It is easier to start thinking of stress in absolute terms, as if there were only two states, stressed or not stressed. In reality, there is a continuum between complete relaxation and utter stress. Stress hormone secretion is not an all or nothing affair. Secretion varies with circumstances.

Cortisol

The ACT hormone message is carried in the blood to the adrenal glands telling them to *release cortisol*. Cortisol releases sugar into the blood from stores in the body to supply energy to muscles which will be needed for action. We secrete cortisol all the time but in varying amounts according to predicted stress and actual stress. Cortisol levels reflect how prepared we are to react to danger in the environment, they mirror our state of arousal. When blood levels are high we are alert, ready to perceive, ready to learn, ready to assess the situation, and ready to act. The degree of arousal reflects the likelihood of behaving instinctively as opposed to behaving purely rationally. The higher the cortisol level, the more aroused we are, and the greater the chance that emotional reactions to situations will predominate over reactions determined by logical reasoning and social conditioning.

The law recognises the distinction between the two types of behaviour, a lesser charge of manslaughter may be brought if a defendant can prove that his actions were unpremeditated, i.e. irrational. Curiously enough the law is one of the few institutions to recognise that a new mother's hormonal state may adversely affect her behaviour; if she kills her baby she is charged with infanticide rather than murder.

Blood levels of cortisol follow a daily rhythm. They are highest at nine in the morning, fall throughout the day and are lowest when we are asleep. This reflects the human lifestyle and reflects the times when we are most likely to encounter danger in the environment – that is, when we are moving around away from home. Nocturnal animals manifest the opposite pattern of cortisol secretion, having their highest levels at night.

One might very well ask whether it might not be better to be prepared for danger at all times. This question is best answered in terms of energy conservation. Being fully alert all the time would cost a lot of energy. Muscles have to be supplied with fuel and oxygen; the heart would need to beat faster; the lungs to take in more oxygen. It is more economical to have a system that uses more power only when necessary; that is during the hours of wakefulness when stressful situations might be predicted; and at times of actual stress. The arousal level stress system is energy efficient. Not only is it efficient because it is tuned to everyday predicted needs, but also because it takes energy away from other body systems concerned with long-term survival – growth, repair and reproduction.

Stress and ß-endorphin

Increased cortisol secretion is accompanied by an increase in another hormone – ß-endorphin. ß-endorphin was discovered relatively recently by researchers looking for a natural opium-like substance in the brain (Kosterlitz and Hughes, 1975). Given that people become so addicted to opium, heroin and morphine, scientists thought that there must be a similar substance occurring naturally within the body. When they found it they called it the endogenous opiate, endorphin or the opium within. There are a number of these substances, ß-endorphin being just one, but it seems to be the most important as far as stress is concerned.

I see ß-endorphin as the link between the mind and the body in stressful situations and also in pregnancy and childbirth; between the behaviour of individual bodily functions and the behaviour of the body as a whole – psychological behaviour.

ß-endorphin

Effects on the mind
- pain relief (a similar effect to morphine, a pain-relieving drug)
- pleasure and euphoria (a similar effect to heroin)
- switches on learning mechanisms
- switches on prolactin, the nest-building hormone

Effects on the body
- slows digestion
- slows some smooth muscle contraction, including reproductive smooth muscle in men and women
- nausea
- dampens down the immune system

Effects on other hormones
- blocks instructions to ovaries
- lowers growth hormone secretion

All these responses are dose related. The more ß-endorphin that is secreted, the stronger the response will be.

ß-endorphin is the main link between mind and body because it has effects on both the mind and the body, all of which have been observed in the stress response and some of which are primary symptoms of pregnancy. The secretion of cortisol by the adrenal glands is the last step in a chain of hormonal messages starting in the brain with the production of a hormone called CRF, corticotrophin releasing factor. The chain reaction that leads to cortisol is: CRF → ACT hormone → cortisol. However, the chain reaction does not just consist of single steps. CRF works by unleashing a group of hormones manufactured in a prohormone string of amino acids – pro-opiomelanocortin (POMC).

In everyday language POMC can be loosely translated as "for opium-like substances, for reactions to light, and for cortisol production." ACT hormone is the section of this long string of hormones that instructs the ad-renal gland to produce cortisol. The other two components are also involved in stress responses. We can forget about the melano/reactions to light section for the moment but the opiate-like substances section of the string is ß-endorphin.

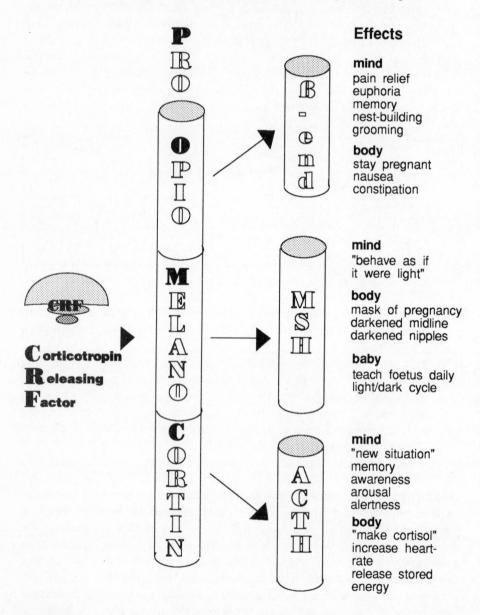

Effects

mind
pain relief
euphoria
memory
nest-building
grooming

body
stay pregnant
nausea
constipation

mind
"behave as if
it were light"

body
mask of pregnancy
darkened midline
darkened nipples

baby
teach foetus daily
light/dark cycle

mind
"new situation"
memory
awareness
arousal
alertness

body
"make cortisol"
increase heart-
rate
release stored
energy

9: POMC

At present the only aspect of ß-endorphin secretion that appears to interest most medical scientists is its effects on pain relief, perhaps because research is often funded by drug companies who are always on the lookout for new pain relievers. However, endocrinologists are now becoming interested in the role of ß-endorphin in regulating secretion of female sex hormones which is again of interest to drug companies because of the large market for contraceptive hormones. There is also interest from doctors working in the field of *in vitro* fertilisation (fertilisation in the test tube). Doctors need to regulate a woman's menstrual cycle for treatment to succeed. This is another area involving large sums of money. None of the research seems to have been directed at understanding normal hormonal control in everyday life.

The ACTION hormones

Stress hormones prepare us for action to change the environment, or our position within it. They switch on instinctive behaviour aimed at making the environment fit our needs better.

We have all been indoctrinated into thinking that stress hormones are bad for us but in fact man needs stress hormones not only to prepare for dangers in the environment but to increase heart rate to enable more blood to reach the brain. For man lack of stress, boredom, is itself a stress – paradoxically relieved by an input of stress. We all know some workaholics who appear to become addicted to stress itself, perhaps they are addicted to ß-endorphin. Perhaps young hooligans also crave the excitement and ß-endorphin that comes from the thrills of outwitting the police – for them the stress caused by the boredom of unemployment is relieved by antisocial behaviour. I suggest that the pleasure effect of ß-endorphin is a psychological reward for seeking out stress, a motivation for avoiding laziness.

Both ACT hormone and ß-endorphin are involved in learning mechanisms. Man has a greater ability to learn than the rest of the animal kingdom, his intelligence results from his increased restlessness. He also needs physically to look for stimulus in his environment to keep his heart pumping against the forces of gravity. The increased need for stress itself may have been the biological route to increased brain power.

Instinctive behaviour turned on by stress hormones has been selected to remove causes of stress, including boredom. In acute stress the instinctive response may be to run away; in less stressful situations the instinctive response may be to modify the environment to make it suit our needs better. If we are unable to act on these instincts then the feeling of being under stress gets worse. Cortisol levels are highest in circumstances of helplessness, hopelessness and lack of control over our environment. Cortisol is secreted when we unable to manipulate our environment to suit ourselves, being forced by circumstances to remain inactive or to act against our instinctive judgements. If we do not act on our instincts, more and more ACT hormone is secreted as our brain tries to nudge us into action to improve our environment. If we are physically unable to manipulate our environment – our stress levels soar. We never become used to having high stress levels, we merely develop coping strategies for living with the situation.

Psychological Stress

Scientists can inflict psychological stress on animals by handling, immobilisation, adding a novel stimulus or a predator to their cages and by making something happen that goes against learned expectations, for example having taught the animal to press a lever for food, experimenters make the action deliver an electric shock instead. Psychological stress can be caused by largely similar methods in humans.

Social pressure

Social animals such as man have more opportunities for experiencing psychological stress simply because their own instinct for self-preservation may run counter to the interests of the group as a whole, and the force of peer pressure makes them act against their instincts and thus causes stress. The reward for altruistic behaviour is social approval, continued acceptance in the social group. The punishment for selfish behaviour is isolation, rejection by the group. A social animal needs the support of the group to survive.

Authority figure pressure

The first authority figure is the mother herself. Simply because she provides the infant with all his needs, she also holds the ultimate sanction against the infant, withdrawal of food itself – which is necessarily accompanied by withdrawal of the breast, physical contact. The next social pressure occurs in the family group. The baby is weaker than all the rest and cannot force other family members to stay with him to provide him with company and stimulation. As he gets older his stronger brothers and sisters as well as his parents can physically force him to conform to their wishes and, since life is more pleasant for him if they play with him, he conforms. As the infant grows more adventurous, this pressure to conform extends to the wider community. Owing to their greater physical strength, adults can reinforce social pressure with bodily sanctions including physical removal from the group and physical punishment for nonconformity. The rewards for conformity are approval and company, the punishments disapproval and social isolation. Parents still threaten naughty children with being put to bed without any supper. Parental pressure is still very powerful and extends to authority figures in adult life from mere force of habit. The disparity in size has now gone, but the psychological pressure remains because of strong conditioning in youth. Respect for authority developed throughout childhood is the foundation for a co-operative society. We are not naturally altruistic but learn to conform through authority pressure. But we want to be accepted into peer groups as well.

Peer pressure

Social animals have an overwhelming need to be part of a group, to conform. Solitary confinement, removal of the prisoner from his peers, is used as a further punishment in prisons. Man is the ultimate social animal in that he participates in all sorts of groups, both formal and informal. Society forms groups covering virtually all aspects of life. People sharing party political, religious, cultural, professional, class and leisure interests club together for the pleasure of each other's society. In all these groups there are enormous pressures to conform or be rejected. Peer pressure is incredibly powerful and the power of the spokesman of the group is greater than the power of the individual wanting change. Nonconformists have always had a hard time of it. The group pressure to resist change proposed by a smaller subsection of the group is very powerful, and the usual result is schism.

Man needs the approval of his peers for his psychological security and it follows that disapproval is stressful. Admittance to groups is behaviour or performance oriented, and tests for admission into a selected group are very stressful. The stress caused by the fear of rejection is so powerful that it can all too easily interfere with performance. Job interviews and examinations are intrinsically stressful and people often know that their performance has not matched their ability. The more one wants to pass the exam or get the job, the greater the fear of rejection and the greater the stress. We inflict stress upon ourselves.

Self-inflicted pressure

The driving test is a classic example of a performance test causing intense psychological stress. It matters not to the driving examiner whether someone passes the test. It matters only to the person himself. Driving tests cause enormous psychological stress because they assess both physical and rational skills at the same time. A driver has to be able to control the pedals to prevent stalling while at the same time he must be aware of and react appropriately to other traffic. Stress hormones interfere with bodily behaviour as well as rational behaviour. The ß-endorphin accompanying psychological stress often makes people nauseous and cortisol supplies muscles with too much energy for the task in hand. The physical response of the body to psychological stress is still a fight or flight reaction, inappropriate for the muscular energy needed to manipulate the controls of a car. By deciding to put in for the test we have already assessed ourselves and decided that we are capable of passing. Failure is humiliating because it questions our ability to predict our own performance, people make many excuses for failure in an attempt to shore up their self-confidence. We often need constant reassurance from other people to restore confidence in ourselves after failure.

Bullying

Bullying is a continual process of belittlement, sapping someone's self-confidence and undermining their position in a group. We need confidence in our own abilities in order to survive and perform well. In the field of education rewarding what is good is seen to be better for a child's self-confidence than punishing mistakes; although failing to point out mistakes may make him over confident and unfitted for the real world where mistakes are punished. Giving a child confidence in one area may improve performance in another. Self-confidence is the hallmark of a successful human being. Lack of confidence leads to underachievement by destroying the very will to succeed. Fear of failure can become so strong that it may spill over into other parts of life and people may become passive and withdraw from society completely.

Stress and depression
If we are stressed and fail to act on our instincts, or fail to improve our environment sufficiently then we risk becoming depressed. High levels of cortisol are accompanied by feelings of helplessness, hopelessness and lack of control over life itself. Depressed people often retreat into themselves and stop even trying to improve their lives but, despite their apparent passivity, their minds are in turmoil and they cannot sleep at night. Depression is a form of learned helplessness and is accompanied by feelings of despair.

Stress and obsessional behaviour
Some obsessional disorders can be explained by effects of ß-endorphin and ACT hormone on memory. During a stressful episode earlier in life, relief from stress may have coincided with some sort of behaviour which, while it was not itself responsible for removing the source of stress, has been subconsciously remembered as if it were. Learning hormones are high during times of stress and, to aid survival, it is as important to remember successful strategies for dealing with stress as it is to remember things that cause stress. At subsequent stressful episodes the same behaviour is hauled out on each occasion when our brain thinks it might be useful. On this model it is easy to see how behaviour such as hand-washing or cleaning up after childhood accidents might have followed a stressful event. It was probably the mother's attention that relieved the stress but, because maternal attention coincided with hand-washing, hand-washing itself became associated with stress relief. In later life hand-washing continues to be hauled out by the subconscious for stress relief whether it is appropriate or not. Because this type of behaviour is the result of conditioning it can be cured in the same way, by behavioural therapy.

Stress in the home
One reason for depression and other psychiatric disorders may be homelessness itself; in the metaphorical sense as well as the literal sense. As children we are subject to authority pressure from parents, but as we grow up we wish to become more independent and we want to rid ourselves of pressure now seen as unnecessary. Many teenagers leave home because they no longer feel at home there. Parents may still treat them as children, which causes psychological stress because it saps self-confidence. Teenagers are also feeling biological urges for procreation and want to make their own home to suit their changing biological needs. Leaving the nest is an indication that people feel ready to be treated as adults. Stress in the home is the worst sort of stress because there is no psychologically safe place for retreat in times of need.

The Biology of Hearth and Home

Nest-building and social behaviour were evolutionary novelties that favoured mammals and birds. Both nest-building and social behaviour can be seen as action taken to improve the physical or psychological environment rather than merely reacting to it. Perhaps mammals fared better than the dinosaurs because they made nests and worked together to improve their environment purposefully. Both nest-building and social behaviour have the same hormonal motivation – prolactin. And prolactin is switched on by ß-endorphin.

Prolactin

Prolactin is named for its physiological role in milk production, it means *for milk*. However, milk production is patently not its only role in life as it is secreted by men as well as women. It is another hormone with a role in both stress and reproduction. It carries two distinct behavioural messages as well as the *make milk* message. It is a hormonal motivation for nest-building behaviour and grooming behaviour. These behaviours are important to reduce physical and psychological stress by improving the environment and making or maintaining friendship. Both activities are designed to remove both actual and predicted stress. When under stress we go home where we feel safe or run to friends for comfort and reassurance. Building a nest is improving the physical environment, making it fit physical needs better. Grooming and being groomed enhances or restores psychological self-confidence.

Nest-building

Prolactin switches on nest-building behaviour in the context of stress and in the context of reproduction. We have a strong need for security. A nest is a place that is an extension of ourselves. The environment of a nest is so familiar that we feel totally at home in it. We can predict the things that are likely to happen in it and only people well known to us will walk through the door without knocking first. Romanies will not let strangers into their caravans at all, their nest is so small that the invasion of privacy feels like physical assault.

Preying animals like lions tend to make nests or lairs in a particular place. For preyed upon animals such as gazelle the herd itself is a kind of mobile social home. Young carnivores can afford to be born unable to walk because they can develop in the safety of a physical nest but young herbivores must be mobile almost at once in order to keep up with the caravan. Home thus can consist of both a fixed place and also the company of friends and relations. Home is a place where one feels at ease, somewhere with little physical or psychological stress. It can be a physical location or a social group.

Grooming

Prolactin switches on grooming behaviour for stress relief and for reproductive purposes. The evolutionary explanation for grooming is that it cements social bonds. Strong social bonds improve the group's chance of survival by leading to co-operative working and sharing resources, a more efficient mode of life that itself leads to spare time for grooming and yet stronger social bonds. Primates in particular spend hours grooming each other; it is a physical reward given for group membership and reassurance of one's position in the group. This is as true for man as it is for other primates. Physical grooming is restricted to sexual partners and family members, but psychological grooming takes place in other groups. Man uses language as well as physical contact for cementing social bonds. Much of our conversation consists of social chat serving no useful purpose except to reinforce group membership. Refusing to talk to people is a way of excluding them from the group.

Grooming is a time-consuming business. But the time is not wasted if it makes us feel good and at the same time encourages the group to work together for the common good. Modern man is often in a hurry, and time is now equated with money. Man has another way of grooming: buying presents to express approval or regain affection. Cats also will bring in "presents" to express approval. The hormonal motivation for grooming behaviour is prolactin and prolactin is switched on by ß-endorphin.

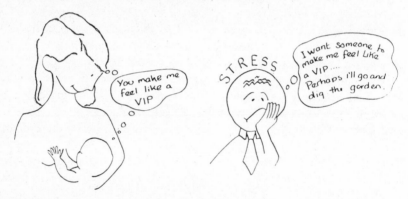

10: Prolactin – A motivation and a reward

Maternal behaviour

Maternal behaviour can be explained almost entirely in terms of nest-building and grooming. Mothers build nests to prepare for birth and groom their children, giving them the present of milk from their own bodies and constantly washing them. For marsupials the very first nest is the mother's own pouch and for other placental mammals the closeness between mother and infants during feeding means that the mother represents the home. Maternal behaviour reduces stress in the infant and rewards the mother who is delighted to have the undivided attention of her babies. Adults have to work to maintain their position in the group but infants are less discriminating in their affections. However, constant grooming is exhausting and infants become more demanding as they grow older. They outgrow their mother's supply of milk and have to be edged out into the wider world to fend for themselves. Prolactin is secreted as a response to birth itself and to being suckled. It is secreted as a response to another hormone, vasointestinal peptide, a hormone associated with eating.

Regulation of prolactin

Prolactin secretion is complicated, reflecting the many different physical and behavioural messages that it carries. Prolactin levels are high at night, low during everyday life and switched on again by the ß-endorphin secretion that accompanies stress. Stress will be relieved by improving the physical environment, nest-building, and by improving the social environment, seeking comfort from friends. Physically stretching the nipples and the vagina switches on prolactin secretion, which accounts for its secretion in sexual intercourse, birth and lactation. Prolactin is thus a mothering hormone promoting behaviour to keep infants physically and psychologically safe.

Human nest-building

Moving house is said to be one of the chief causes of stress in life. When we move house we are abandoning much that is familiar and having to start again in a new place, with different neighbours and different routines. At least our possessions remain the same and they assume a special importance to modern itinerant man – the ubiquitous motor car acquires a special significance as a nest on wheels. People literally see their cars as an extension of themselves and motorists are notoriously quick to defend the territory of their car.

When we move house ACT hormone, ß-endorphin, cortisol and prolactin are secreted in greater quantities because we lose the security of our old nest; we nest-build with a madness born of the need to recreate a safe haven as a buffer against the unpredictability of the outside world. People who have been burgled feel violated by the thought that someone has disturbed the sanctity of their home; it never feels quite so safe again.

Paradoxically, the modern craze for moving house every few years is a direct result of too much stress in our life. We think that life would be better if only we could change our surroundings and move, or add a conservatory, or refit the kitchen – the advertising industry plays on these basic instincts. However, life is not much better following these improvements, because the underlying causes of stress are not removed, and so the stress cycle goes on. The underlying causes can be many and varied – poor family relationships, overwork, boredom, lack of creative outlets and so on.

Both boredom and overwork can lead to depression and some people try to spend their way out of depression but the stress-relieving effects of spending tend to be short-lived. Do-it-yourself, craft, sewing, cooking and gardening are far better ways of relieving stress as they are physical activities, and we feel a real sense of creative achievement on seeing the results of our own labour. Physical nest-building dissipates stress and restlessness. The improvements wrought merely by spending money are less likely to lead to any lasting psychological benefit.

Economics of nest-building

Prolactin equals money for the capitalist. Western economic strategies are founded on the need to maintain growth by increasing consumption – our grandmother's saucepans probably lasted all her life, but we tend to replace

69

them when they become worn; saucepans are no longer even designed to last a lifetime. Built-in obsolescence is a fundamental requirement of a society that depends on increased consumption for its survival. High stress levels in the developed world directly cause an escalating consumption of the world's resources, both renewable and non-renewable. The bill is paid today by third world citizens who receive a pittance for their work and raw materials. The debt must also be repaid tomorrow by our own descendants. Western economies are rooted in maintaining high stress levels to generate consumption; advertising is a way of increasing stress artificially by playing on instincts, which should instead be stress removing activities, and thus generating dissatisfaction.

A situation where consumer demand is falling has dire consequences for a monetarist economy. The economic recession of the 1990s has been directly attributed to the depression of the housing market. Overall economic activity fell because fewer people moved house and therefore had no need to fill the new house with the myriad bits and pieces purchased to personalise one's home. This led to a downward spiral leading to bankruptcies and job losses in all sectors of the economy, with the exception of health insurance.

Although people are stressed by fear of unemployment, the fear of losing one's home altogether is enough to make people save instead of spend. Problems in the housing market are literally too close to home to allow any easy recovery.

Even the medical take-over of childbirth can be viewed from this economic angle. Despite the fact that childbirth is safer now than it has ever been because more of us are closer to achieving our genetic potential, professionals play on the fear instinct to coerce women into hospital birth and thus increase consumption of hospital services and safeguard their own jobs, wittingly or unwittingly. Fear of childbirth is still the biggest hurdle to be overcome, despite Dick-Read's pioneering work of sixty years ago.

Nest-building in pregnancy

We feel the urge to build a nest when we no longer feel at peace with our surroundings because we are stressed. However, women have the nest-building urge when they are enjoying a peaceful and happy pregnancy. The consumer society plays on this urge into promoting more and more baby equipment at escalating prices. Pregnant women need to build a nest to prepare for their child and to prepare for a radically new change of lifestyle – the onset of motherhood. They are also unwittingly preparing the home for labour itself because labour proceeds more smoothly in stress-free surroundings.

A nest for labour

Nature intended labour to take place at home among friends, in a place of safety where stress levels are low: where the world is predictable, where the surroundings are familiar, where intruders are not welcomed except by invitation, where the residents control the environment, and where the stranger abides by the rules of the house or is turned out. All other mammals choose to find a safe place in which to labour because stress hormones are intricately involved in labour. Why should woman be an exception?

Hospital birth

Western woman goes to hospital to have her baby for two reasons. First because she has been taught by society that hospital birth is safer than home birth, and second because she thinks that she will be looked after better in hospital. Both of these assumptions are false. Hospital birth turns what should be like an ordinary car journey into a situation resembling a driving test. Labour is a high performance task when body and mind have to work together for the best result. Authority figure pressure, peer pressure and pressure from oneself all lead to higher secretion of stress hormones which interfere with labour. Social pressure to give birth in hospital saps self-confidence before labour even starts.

Hospital can never be home and stress hormone production must increase to cope with the intense psychological stress of hospital. The nest-building instinct is one of the few instincts acknowledged by medical textbooks and yet its implications are totally ignored. Even a sympathetic GP may say with one breath, "So you're frantically nest-building, are you?" and with the next, "Have you made arrangements for the other children for when you're in hospital?"

We choose baby equipment, wallpaper the nursery, spring clean the house and create the right environment for the baby. Then we leave it all behind at the first signs of labour and rush to hospital, worrying whether we will get there in time, worrying about the children we have left behind, wondering whether there will be anyone on duty that we know in the hospital – and sending our stress hormone levels sky high. Sometimes so high that we are sent home again and have to go through the whole rigmarole all over again at a later date.

3 Stress and Reproduction

" A paradox, a paradox, a most ingenious paradox"
Gilbert and Sullivan in *The Pirates of Penzance*

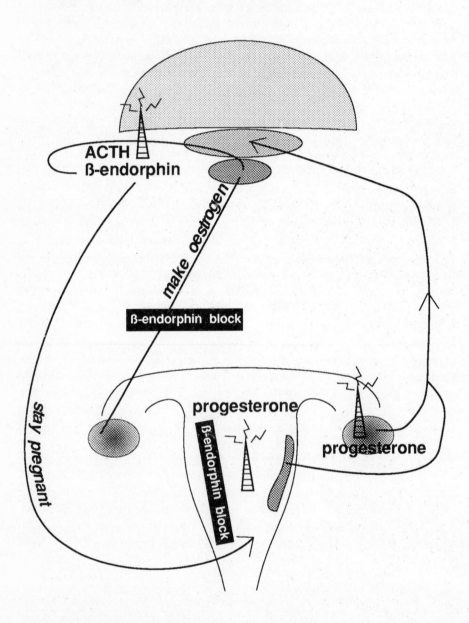

11: Stress hormones in pregnancy

Stress hormones are deeply involved in reproduction. At the same time, they interfere with it. ß-endorphin prevents the uterus rejecting the foreign body of the foetus and placenta unit by reducing the immune response and by preventing expulsive uterine contractions, both of which are the body's normal response to a foreign body. Prolactin switches on maternal behaviour. Progesterone, the steroid hormone that is actually named for its central role in pregnancy, "for gestation", switches on another hormonal route for ß-endorphin secretion (Olster and Blaustein, 1990). Progesterone therefore increases ß-endorphin secretion. ß-endorphin secretion inhibits maternal oestrogen production (Laatikainen, 1991). ß-endorphin regulates the secretion of the labour hormone, oxytocin and switches on prolactin. Progesterone and pregnancy itself gives women naturally higher levels of stress hormones. Cortisol levels in pregnant women are six times higher than in non-pregnant women. Higher than normal stress hormone levels are needed to maintain pregnancy. Levels may be raised even higher by psychological stress. Both prolonged (chronic) and short-term (acute) psychological stress have also been found to play a role in infertility, miscarriage and premature labour (Shaarawy et al, 1991; Läpple, 1988; Omer and Everly, 1988). Pregnancy and labour are physical stresses and we should expect to find increased stress hormones in pregnant and labouring women.

Stress, fertilisation and implantation
Fertilisation itself may depend on an optimum level of stress hormones in the blood during a particular time in the menstrual cycle. High ß-endorphin levels can block ovulation so that no egg is available for fertilisation and low progesterone and ß-endorphin levels can prevent implantation.

Technology's answer to infertility owed to stress-induced anovulation is sometimes to pile on yet more stress by attempting in vitro fertilisation, an invasive hospital treatment that causes physiological stress on top of pre-existing psychological stress. This has to be a totally mad way to treat infertility and it is not surprising that the failure rate of IVF is around 80-90%. The first treatment for infertility caused by high stress levels should be simple advice to take up stress-reducing activities, for example, meditation or yoga. Biofeedback techniques for reducing mental stress are now available and these could be tried before subjecting women to the added stress of infertility treatment. There may even be a simple drug treatment for infertility. Naloxone, a drug that counteracts the effects of morphine and ß-endorphin, has been found to induce ovulation in animals but "the effects on fertility are unknown" (Laatikainen, 1991). This might seem a sensible treatment for women whose infertility is caused by failure to ovulate owing to high stress levels caused by infertility itself, a vicious circle.

Miscarriage and premature labour
High levels of stress hormones can reduce progesterone levels and thus, paradoxically, reduce overall stress hormone levels. Progesterone is one step in the metabolic pathway for making other steroid hormones such as testosterone,

the aggression hormone. Although testosterone is thought of as a male hormone because it is manufactured in the testes, women may also need to act aggressively to survive. They produce testosterone in the adrenal gland which can produce all steroid hormones. Reduced progesterone will lead to reduced ß-endorphin secretion which may lead to miscarriage or premature labour. If a pregnant woman is in a very dangerous situation she can fight for survival by cutting off ß-endorphin supplies to her foetus. Nature, like doctors, will prefer to save a mother's life if there is a choice to be made. The explanation for this is simple. The mother has already reached her childbearing years, nature regards her as a bird in the hand and knows that she can have another baby. The foetus is only worth two in the bush. It has a long road to travel before it can pass on its genes. Moreover, a dead pregnant mother means a dead foetus.

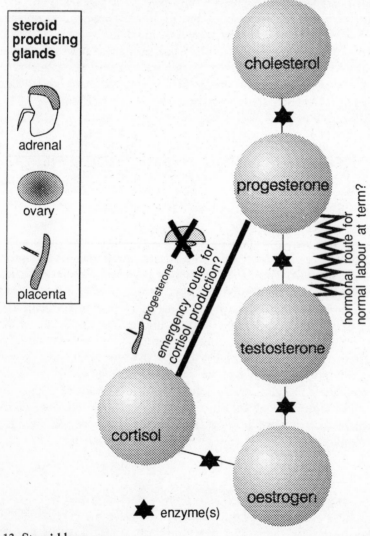

12: Steroid hormones

In premature labour, high maternal stress can raise stress hormones levels in the amniotic fluid (the waters) and, since high foetal stress hormone levels are probably the mechanism that causes normal labour at term (Goland *et al*, 1988), high levels earlier in pregnancy may precipitate premature labour.

Women whose work leads to higher secretion of stress hormones – those working at the two ends of the work spectrum, doing heavy manual work or boring work, and those with high pressure jobs – are far more likely to have premature deliveries and weaker babies (Homer *et al*, 1990).

Reproduction and stress are linked together in all these ways because the environment is all important for birth and mothering. A woman has relatively few chances to give birth and bring up children compared to mammals having large litters several times a year. She is pregnant for nine long months at a time and then must nurture the child intensively for at least another year. It is important that she does not waste reproductive time conceiving and carrying babies that have a poor chance of survival to adulthood owing to a poor environment and poor maternal support system. There are selective advantages in miscarrying even normal babies if a mother is under too much stress. If she miscarries, she can spend energy on putting her environment to rights before trying again, rather than trying to nurture a foetus at the same time. This seems to be another paradox. Prolactin, the environment changing hormone, is high both in stress and in pregnancy. If a woman has the energy needed for building a special nest for labour and mothering, why is there not enough energy for stress-relieving behaviour? Perhaps the stressed pregnant female has to exert twice as much effort making a physical and social environment that is secure for her and also secure for her future family.

ß-endorphin in normal pregnancy

Levels of ß-endorphin are so high in pregnancy that, in the early days of research in the 1970s, it was thought that it was only secreted during pregnancy (Suda *et al*, 1978). However, techniques for measuring blood levels have improved and it is now known that levels fluctuate during the menstrual cycle, increasing with rising progesterone secretion in the second half of the cycle and decreasing with falling progesterone secretion at menstruation. ß-endorphin regulates sex steroid production and blocks expulsive uterine contractions. When the block is removed menstruation or labour ensue. It seems rather paradoxical that stress hormone levels should be higher in pregnant women but the reasons become clearer when one considers the needs of the pregnant woman and her foetus.

Freedom from restlessness and a pregnancy "high"

Pregnancy is very demanding on the mother's body. Women have to provide, through their own blood, everything that the foetus needs to survive and mature. They have to manufacture more blood and their heart has to work harder. They have to carry around a lot more weight and yet they need to rest more in order to concentrate energy resources on the foetus. Pregnant women are therefore, I think, relieved of mankind's natural urge for constant mental stimulation to produce cortisol to keep the heart pumping adequately in the upright position. Progesterone, the pregnancy hormone, switches on a new pathway for producing heart-maintaining stress hormones. Cortisol levels in pregnant women are six times higher than normal and yet pregnant women are not six times as stressed by the environment. On the contrary, pregnant women often feel more placid, peaceful and even euphoric.

This mental state is typical of high ß-endorphin levels. The opiate "high" of pregnancy may be a natural reward for being pregnant. At the same time pregnant women are notorious for their heightened emotionality. High stress hormone levels increase arousal and therefore increase the chance of an emotional response to a situation as opposed to a more "rational" response (but see p.135). Many people are aware of the need to treat pregnant women with kid gloves, sparing them bad news, and trying to relieve them from unnecessary stress. Advice to expectant fathers nearly always contains a section on the expectant mother's changed moods (Parsons, 1975; Bourne, 1989).

Physical effects

ß-endorphin has profound influences on the immune system (Plotnikoff and Murgo, 1985) and stops smooth muscle contracting (Kosterlitz and Hughes, 1975). In pregnancy a woman needs both these actions of ß-endorphin in her womb. The uterus has to contain and nurture the foreign bodies of the foetus and placenta, both of which are made up of different genetic material which the body would normally reject. The natural response of the immune system to a foreign body is to expel it. For example, organ transplant specialists have to give very powerful drugs to stop the body rejecting transplanted organs made up of foreign genetic material. Levels of ß-endorphin found in the blood in the first trimester of pregnancy are high enough to account for the constipation and nausea of early pregnancy. In the first few weeks ß-endorphin is produced by the mother's hypothalamus as a response to progesterone from the corpus luteum (the part of the ovary from whence the egg came). Nausea is far more common in the morning when circadian stress hormone levels are high and when stress-induced ß-endorphin is secreted on top of pregnancy-induced ß-endorphin.

Other sources of ß-endorphin

But not all ß-endorphin is produced by the mother herself. As the placenta and foetal membranes get larger they secrete significant quantities. Pregnancy places such an enormous stress on the mother that if it were left to her body to decide whether to continue with the pregnancy or to miscarry her body would probably reject its parasite. So she is not given the chance to decide for herself.

Once the foetus and placenta are big enough to start causing problems by using up too much maternal energy, they produce ß-endorphin themselves. ß-endorphin is produced by the placenta and the foetal membranes. But this foeto-placental ß-endorphin is produced locally, in the uterus, and used locally,

76

in the uterus, a hormonal action known as paracrine action. During pregnancy the ovaries also secrete ß-endorphin.

Once the placenta takes over progesterone production and can manufacture ß-endorphin for itself, between the eighth and twelfth week of pregnancy, maternally produced ß-endorphin can fall without risk of miscarriage, and morning sickness becomes less of a problem. This changeover time for ß-endorphin production is around the time when miscarriages are most common because maternally produced ß-endorphin may fall before the placenta is producing enough to maintain pregnancy. Maternal blood ß-endorphin has been observed by some researchers to fall in the middle trimester (Browning et al, 1983). But it must not fall completely – some is still needed at the hypothalamus to stop the mother's ovaries from regaining control of oestrogen production.

Stress and Problems in Pregnancy

ß-endorphin secretion seems to need to be finely tuned for each stage of pregnancy. Too much and the pregnancy may miscarry, and too little and the pregnancy may miscarry. Given that pregnant women have naturally high stress hormone levels, any further increase caused by psychological stress itself will be likely to cause problems. High maternal stress can distress the foetus and trigger premature labour, but the foetus does not always respond in the most appropriate way for the mother – by giving the signal for birth and bringing to an end the stress of pregnancy. Pre-eclampsia, or pregnancy induced hypertension (high blood pressure) is an indication that maternal stress hormone levels are becoming dangerously high. Bedrest is given in an attempt to contain the problem of pre-eclampsia but the only cure is delivery. Eclampsia itself is life-threatening for the mother and foetus and its physical and mental effects which include heart failure and hallucinations could be owed to a natural overdose of ß-endorphin. At present this theory is mere speculation, but it would be easy to test by prescribing naloxone, a competitor for ß-endorphin receptors in cell membranes, for experimentally induced pre-eclampsia in animals.

The older name for eclampsia is toxaemia which implies that doctors once suspected it to be caused by a toxin. The main clinical sign of pre-eclampsia is raised blood pressure. But it has been shown that place of blood pressure measurement affects actual blood pressure. Blood pressure is raised in stressful circumstances and is nearly always lower when measured at home. Differences can be quite startling. My own blood pressure used to rise by 20 points when measured in the consultant's clinic. Hospital antenatal clinics can themselves fill some antenatal beds unnecessarily. Women who are advised to have their labour induced because of high blood pressure are well advised to request a home blood pressure reading before committing themselves to perhaps needless intervention. A woman whose blood pressure level is always raised in hospital antenatal clinics should seriously consider having her baby at home because high stress levels prolongs labour and the more stress a woman feels in a hospital setting the more likely it is that she will have problems if she labours in hospital.

Stress hormones balance the biological needs of mother and foetus.
Pregnancy, birth and mothering represent an enormous investment in time and energy on the part of the mother. If it were not for the joy that children bring to their parents and the basic biological urge to reproduce, no woman in her right mind would choose to become a mother. Pregnancy and childbirth also put the mother at a greater risk of death, despite the best efforts of natural selection towards safer childbirth. Yet women become pregnant and put up with the physiological stress of pregnancy and, moreover, go through the whole process again and again. The need for children more than compensates for the stresses of pregnancy. ß-endorphin produced by the mother, her ovaries, the placenta and the foetal membranes, maintains pregnancy. Genes for making sure of the survival of the species (Richard Dawkin's "selfish" genes) overrule genes for the survival of the individual woman. Stress hormones in pregnancy and reproduction are therefore also concerned with survival; but instead of favouring short-term survival of the individual over long-term survival of the individual, this time they favour long-term survival of the species over long-term survival of the individual.

Other hormonal effects in pregnancy
In the previous chapter it was stated that ACT hormone and ß-endorphin are secreted in conjunction with another hormone – MSH, melanocyte stimulating hormone, or "response to light" hormone. Higher than usual levels of MSH in pregnant women lead to changes in body colour: a dark line develops down the midline of the body, nipples often become darker, and sometimes women's faces darken slightly and show the aptly named *mask of pregnancy*. I think the biological purpose of this hormone may be to teach the foetus a daily cycle of light and dark. The foetus is largely deprived of light cues when in the womb but yet is born showing a circadian rhythm of cortisol secretion. Effects on skin colour are therefore a side effect on the mother in the same way that morning sickness and constipation are a side effect of raised ß-endorphin.

Oestrogens
Oestrogens are manufactured mainly in the ovaries and the placenta. They develop and maintain the female reproductive organs, they promote growth of the breasts and they regulate the menstrual cycle. They also increase the number of carrier molecules for cortisol in the blood. In pregnancy, oestrogens prepare the uterus for labour by linking together individual uterine muscle fibres; forming electrical gap junctions between cells so that, in labour, uterine muscle fibre activity can be co-ordinated and contractions can spread throughout the uterus as a whole. Oestrogens are also responsible for making the uterus more sensitive to adrenaline, the sudden stress hormone released from the blood from the adrenal glands and acting on nerve cells. Oestrogens are important in enabling the body to take calcium from food. This calcium is need for the formation of bone by the foetus and also for the uterine muscle

which needs calcium to work – to contract and relax. The placenta produces more oestrogen towards the end of pregnancy, acting on instructions from the foetus which provides a necessary substance (substrate) from which the placenta manufactures oestrogen. There is also some evidence that the mother's ovaries resume oestrogen manufacture at the end of pregnancy.

High levels of oestrogen are needed for labour to start and proceed normally. Oestrogen removes the ß-endorphin block on the uterus which, I suggest, maintains pregnancy. Oestrogen and ß-endorphin compete for the same hormone receptors at the hypothalamus (Vertes, Pamer and Garai, 1986) and perhaps at the uterus itself.

This putative role of maternal oestrogen in the onset of labour is contentious but it is supported by research on pregnant rats (Devorshak-Harvey, 1988) and Rhesus monkeys near term (Figuero *et al*, 1989). The rats were found to resume LH secretion (the *make oestrogen* message) at night and the monkeys were more responsive to contraction-promoting hormones at night. Traditionally we think that the onset of human labour is also at night, a time when cortisol levels and thus ACT hormone and ß-endorphin levels are low. Medical science says that births are spread out evenly throughout the day and night, but *time of onset of labour* does not seem to have been considered. Moreover, as most births now take place in hospital and hospitals are better staffed during the day, present figures on time of birth are more likely to reflect current clinical practice rather than nature's clock. Labour is unlikely to be induced at 5 p.m. but likely to be accelerated so that babies are born before the end of the working day.

Progesterone

Progesterone is found in non-mammals but has no particular hormonal job to do, it is merely a precursor to other steroid hormones which include cortisol, oestrogen and testosterone. But at some stage in evolution it started to have an effect on reproduction and gradually acquired a central role in maintaining pregnancy and preparing the body for childbearing and childcare. Progesterone tricks the uterus into thinking itself pregnant by switching on ß-endorphin. This is how the progesterone birth control pill works. The physiological state of the uterus depends more on hormonal influences than the presence or absence of a foetus. Sometimes the foetus dies *in utero* but is not expelled because the placenta may continue to secrete progesterone. Sometimes the placenta continues to develop in the absence of a foetus.

Perhaps the very first effect of progesterone in mammals was a simple delay in the expulsion of eggs – females that incubated their eggs in their bodies for just a little longer left more offspring than those who expelled their eggs earlier. Whatever the first step, this novel use of progesterone has had far reaching effects amongst which are: preventing expulsive contractions of the uterus during pregnancy; inhibiting milk production until the child is born; and preparing for labour by increasing receptors for oestrogen and stimulating maternal aggressiveness.

It is interesting to note that some researchers have found a link between progesterone and intelligence (Dalton, 1984). Progestogens (synthetic progesterone) were sometimes used to prevent miscarriage and mothers given this treatment before the sixteenth week of pregnancy were found to have more intelligent children. Progesterone itself may have been a route to the increased intelligence that gave early mammals such an advantage over the dinosaurs. Given the links between progesterone and ß-endorphin, and ß-endorphin and learning this seems a likely explanation for the acquisition of intelligence.

The main source of progesterone in early pregnancy is the corpus luteum, the follicle from which the egg was released. However, the placenta, which is controlled by the foetus, takes over most progesterone production between the sixth and ninth week of pregnancy. Abortion can be procured by administering an anti-progesterone drug RU486.

Progesterone is a fundamental requirement for the maintenance of pregnancy but, in humans, does not seem to block labour itself. In many animals a fall in progesterone signals the onset of labour. But while for some women, progesterone levels fall towards the end of pregnancy, in others progesterone levels remain high until labour has already started. The ratio of progesterone to oestrogen is more important than the actual quantities. Moreover, the site from which samples are taken may lead to different results. Blood taken from the arm may have a very different ratio of the two hormones than amniotic fluid (Romero *et al*, 1988).

Progesterone also blocks milk production, depressing the milk ejecting hormone, oxytocin. Progesterone-induced ß-endorphin blocks oxytocin release. Milk is secreted within hours of birth in mammals whose labour starts with a fall in progesterone but women secrete only colostrum for the first few days after birth. I suspect that women need the effects of progesterone right up until labour starts because bipedalism puts a greater strain on the cervical end of the uterus in women than it does in quadrupeds.

Testosterone

Conversion of progesterone into testosterone may be part of the hormonal route to normal labour at term. (See figure 12 p 74) There is a rise in female testosterone levels immediately before labour. The physiological purpose of female testosterone is to increase physical stamina to cope with labour and the psychological role is to increase maternal aggression to enable the mother to protect herself during labour and to protect her child after the birth. Women nearing labour may be "uppity", more assertive and aggressive than they normally are, and this may cause problems in communication with professionals.

Development of the Foetal Endocrine System

Almost as soon as the sex hormone secreting glands, the gonads, are formed, they start to secrete sex hormones which act on the developing foetus to produce a phenotypical male or female. The male sex hormone, androgen, must be secreted and taken up by the body tissues to produce a male foetus. In the absence of androgen, or when the tissues lack receptor sites for androgens, a female body will ensue. The default mechanism is female. A genetic male will develop female characteristics if deprived of androgen *in utero*. The hormonal environment of the foetus *in utero* also affects behaviour. Female rat foetuses who are sandwiched between two male foetuses will develop more aggressive, male behaviour after birth than female rat foetuses surrounded by females *in utero*.

The mother's hormones also influence the foetus. On the whole, the foetal liver is very good at screening out maternal hormones received via the umbilical cord but mistakes can happen: male foetuses whose mothers were highly stressed in pregnancy tend to have reduced levels of androgens and, despite male genitals, may show a reduction in male type behaviour after birth – maternal corticosteroids can affect foetal androgens. There is two-way traffic of hormones from the mother to the placenta and foetus and vice versa. Mother and foetus influence each other's behaviour by exchanging hormones. If the mother has a surge of adrenaline the foetus responds by kicking. Numerous examples of this type of reciprocal behaviour can be found in *The Secret Life of the Unborn Child* (Verny and Kelly, 1981).

Foetal stress hormones
The foetus must be protected from high levels of maternal cortisol which would impede growth by switching off growth hormone. Cortisol and other stress hormones switch behaviour of both body and mind from growth, repair and reproduction to short-term survival. The membranes inactivate most maternal cortisol but perhaps cannot deal with very high levels (Murphy, 1979). The environmental influences causing small-for-dates babies are well documented and can be accounted for by maternal stress, both physiological and psychological, leading to foetal stress and cutting off growth hormone.

Stress hormones and the onset of labour
Life in the womb must be gloriously uncomplicated for the foetus. There is no need to worry about where the next meal will come from or how to keep warm. Yet at some point in pregnancy the foetus chooses to be born and to come to terms with the stresses of life outside the womb. This time is usually determined by the maturation of the foetal stress hormone system. The foetus is ready to be born when its hormonal system has developed sufficiently to cope with life outside the womb – where the environment is radically different from the environment of the uterus. Birth itself will necessarily impose a large amount of stress on the foetus; it will be pounded by the forces of uterine contractions and squeezed through a narrow passage, its blood supply will be disrupted by contractions and by the constriction of the umbilical cord against the mother's vagina. The foetus needs to be able to respond appropriately in order to survive birth. High levels of ACT hormone, ß-endorphin and cortisol are found in babies whose mothers deliver them spontaneously at term.

It is easy to see foetal stress purely in a negative light, but a well developed foetal stress response to environmental change is a fundamental requirement for a safe birth and a smooth transition to the outside world. The baby who is ready to react and adapt to a new environment is the baby who is likely to survive the trauma of birth and expulsion from the haven of the womb.

Babies are born with a circadian rhythm of cortisol secretion and there is evidence that time of birth affects perinatal mortality. Babies born at nine in the morning when cortisol levels are at their highest are more likely to survive than those born in the afternoon when circadian cortisol levels have fallen (Rose, 1988). The baby needs high stress hormone levels to survive birth – the greatest shock to the system that there can be.

I really cannot refrain from pointing out that the usual clinical practice of inducing labour at nine in the morning, in an effort to make sure that the baby is born during office hours when staff are available, will inevitably give the induced baby a worse start in life than could be otherwise achieved. An induced baby is already at risk of prematurity and respiratory distress and is also disadvantaged by virtue of the clinical reason for the induction – if a clinical reason exists at all. Perhaps maternity hospitals should start their day at one in the morning if they want to make sure that labour lasts the standard eight hours.

Length of pregnancy is usually dictated by the normal development of the foetal stress hormone system. Labour is preceded by a steep rise in ACT hormone releasing factor (CRF) in the foetus and hence a rise in foetal stress hormones which include cortisol and ß-endorphin. The foetus indicates its readiness to be born when it is capable of surviving outside the womb. Rising ACT hormone levels place it on full alert to prepare it for a radical change in the environment.

Cortisol and lung maturity

As far as the foetus is concerned, the biggest challenge at birth is the change from receiving oxygen from his mother's blood via the placenta, to obtaining his oxygen supply from his own lungs. This time is determined chiefly by lung maturity, which scientists have observed to correlate closely with rising cortisol levels (Mendelson and Boggaram, 1990). Before birth foetal lungs are like collapsed balloons and they need to be expanded as fully as possible to maximise the amount of oxygen going into the blood stream from the very first breath; breathing must be established by the fourth minute after birth or the baby will become brain damaged. At birth, for a short time, the new born baby receives oxygen from both his mother, via the pulsating umbilical cord, and from his lungs; but blood supply to the cord is soon cut off by the contracting uterus to prevent the mother from haemorrhaging to death, so the child soon has to rely on his own efforts.

Efficient lung function depends on the ability of the lungs to expand fully. Lungs are lined with surfactant, a substance that stops the internal walls sticking together and thus allows the lungs to expand to their fullest. Lung surfactant production requires foetal cortisol. The foetus must gain its supplies of cortisol for lung surfactant manufacture from its own adrenal glands because nearly all the cortisol reaching him from his mother is converted by the placenta or membranes into an inactive substance (Murphy, 1979). When the foetus is making enough cortisol it can make enough lung surfactant and is ready to be born.

Premature babies often suffer from respiratory distress syndrome (RDS) which is caused by a relative lack of lung surfactant – various bits of the lung balloons stay stuck together instead of expanding, this reduces the amount of air in the lungs and consequently the amount of oxygen available to the blood. The stress to the foetus of birth itself increases the manufacture of cortisol and thus lung surfactant. Babies born by caesarean section are deprived of this additional cortisol and are thus more likely to suffer RDS. If they have been delivered by elective caesarean section before the mother has laboured normally at all, they are doubly deprived of hormones necessary for efficient lung function. Yet, according to some obstetricians, "There are no contraindications for caesarean section."

It is becoming standard obstetric practice to try to provide the foetus with cortisol for lung maturation but it is difficult to do this by giving cortisol via the mother because the membranes inactivate cortisol. It has been suggested that cortisol could be put into amniotic fluid for the foetus to swallow.

ß-endorphin at the placenta

During pregnancy ß-endorphin manufacture is likely to result from the *make ß-endorphin* message carried by progesterone but near term this message is carried by ACT hormone releasing factor (CRF) instead (Margioris *et al*, 1988). For birth itself the placenta must protect the foetal blood supply even more from the forces of uterine contractions. It steps up production of ß-endorphin and ACT hormone, both of which protect that part of the uterus touching it from contracting.

The foetal blood also adds more ß-endorphin and ACT hormone to the placenta, so the uterus at the placental site is shielded from contractions even more. Once the baby is breathing by himself, he no longer needs the placenta and rejects it by cutting off the supplies of ß-endorphin that go direct to the placenta, thereby removing its part of the placental block.

Maternal Factors in the Onset of Labour

During pregnancy, the uterus is dominated by ß-endorphin supplied by the action of progesterone at the placenta and the ovaries. High levels of ß-endorphin in the brain stop the ovaries from secreting oestrogen. When brain levels drop, the *make oestrogen* message is sent to the ovaries and they secrete oestrogen and wire up the uterus ready for labour. I think that it is the oestrogen/ß-endorphin ratio that is important in the onset of labour rather than the oestrogen/progesterone ratio. Of course a changing ratio of oestrogen/progesterone would cause a changing oestrogen/ß-endorphin ratio because progesterone increases ß-endorphin manufacture.

Labour can start when increased foetal stress hormones provide the signal to the mother that the foetus is ready for birth. However, the rising foetal stress hormone message cannot be sufficient in itself to initiate labour, or postmaturity would be unheard of. Some babies show definite signs of postmaturity: they have started to lose body fat that would have nourished them for the first few days of life before the mother's milk came in; the bones of their heads have become harder and less able to mould to pass through the birth canal. What is it that turns a protective, pregnant womb into a labouring expulsive uterus? Oestrogen.

Oestrogen prepares the uterus for labour

Oestrogen changes the mechanical nature of uterine tissue from contraction resistant to contraction promoting. Oestrogen makes electrical links (gap junctions) between individual muscle cells of the uterus – it wires up the uterus to work as a whole as it needs to during labour.

Human placentas do not contain the right ingredients for oestrogen manufacture. In order to make oestrogen the placenta needs to obtain the raw material for oestrogen manufacture from the foetus (Conley and Mason, 1990). Towards the end of pregnancy the foetus supplies more of this ingredient and oestrogen levels rise in the placenta – another signal from the foetus that it is getting ready to be born.

Throughout pregnancy, the mother's sex hormone system has been taken over by the placenta. In women who are not pregnant the hypothalamus and pituitary gland control the production of oestrogen by the ovaries, but a pregnant woman secretes hardly any LH, the *make oestrogen* message. Progesterone has filtered through the placenta to the mother's blood and turned on ß-endorphin at her hypothalamus which has stopped release of LH. (See figure 11 on p?) This is the same method used to block ovulation, and pregnant women do not need to ovulate for the duration of pregnancy. During pregnancy the ovaries are controlled not by the mother but by the placenta, genetically part of the foetus. They manufacture ß-endorphin and ACT hormone, both of which prevent the co-ordinated uterine contractions of labour.

The uterus needs to be wired up for labour. Oestrogen wires up the uterus and the ovaries manufacture oestrogen. It would seem logical to assume that the placenta stops sending the progesterone *make ß-endorphin/stop oestrogen* message to the mother's hypothalamus, thereby giving her back control over her ovaries, and initiating a surge of maternal oestrogen. We know that the placenta produces CRF which also promotes ß-endorphin manufacture. Perhaps the placenta produces CRF *instead of* progesterone in mammals whose labour starts with falling progesterone levels. Progesterone is a small steroid molecule that can pass freely into the maternal blood but CRF is a large molecule and tends to be used near its source. Neither ß-endorphin nor CRF can cross the placenta. At present this is mere speculation but it fits the hormonal facts as far as they are known. A progesterone primed uterus cannot contract as a whole as it must during labour unless it has been wired up by oestrogen (Csapo, 1966). The uterus needs oestrogen from both the placenta and, I suggest, the ovaries to function effectively in labour.

Onset of labour can be delayed when, despite being allowed to regain control of her sex hormone system, the mother fails to tell her ovaries to manufacture oestrogen and thus complete the wiring up of the uterus. What can stop the mother from instructing her ovaries to produce oestrogen? Stress.

Stress and the onset of labour

Just as high stress levels can stop a woman from ovulating – releasing an egg – high stress levels can prevent a woman from releasing her baby. High brain (maternally produced) ß-endorphin blocks the message to the ovaries to release oestrogen. The baby does not, I think, have total control over the timing of his birth. Evolution, while not allowing her to decide when to start to labour, has given the mother the right of veto over the foetal and placental instructions that the baby is ready to be born by continuing to cut off maternal oestrogen.

While obstetricians claim that births take place at random throughout the day, I believe that the onset of labour depends on maternal ß-endorphin levels. My own research, looking at records of thirty-six women having home births, has shown that only four of them called the midwife between 9 a.m. and 4 p.m. The vast majority called the midwife in the late afternoon or during the night, that is when circadian stress hormones were low or falling. This supports the ß-endorphin block hypothesis. In an older study, researchers found that ACT hormone levels in maternal blood related to the length of labour (Kauppila and Tuimala, 1974).

ß-endorphin and oestrogen are hormonal competitors – they compete with each other for receptor sites in cells (Vertes *et al*, 1986). ß-endorphin "jams" oestrogen receiving stations. If this happens at the level of the brain the LH *make oestrogen* message from the mother's hypothalamus fails to reach her pituitary gland and thus her ovaries. If this happens also at the level of the uterus, as I believe it will be found to do, then the onset of labour will depend on which hormone is winning the fight for cell receptor occupation. While ß-endorphin predominates the uterus cannot be wired up for labour, but when oestrogen starts to predominate then labour will gradually start.

The onset of labour is gradual. Gradually the cervix ripens and becomes soft and stretchy, and gradually muscles cells are linked together by electrical connections to allow Braxton Hicks co-ordinated contractions to spread and involve the whole uterus instead of subsiding again without spreading as they do in late pregnancy. Gradually the uterus comes to be dominated by oestrogen instead of ß-endorphin.

Cervical ripening

Even before the uterus is wired up by oestrogen the door of the uterus, the cervix, must be unlocked. Prostaglandins, locally produced paracrine hormones, "ripen" the cervix and prostaglandins are also part of the natural healing system of the body, the immune system. In his book *Primal Health* Dr Michel Odent blames stress, a poorly developed immune system and reduced prostaglandin production for the diseases of civilisation – among which can be included postmaturity. ß-endorphin reduces the immune response in times of stress. One researcher has suggested that ß-endorphin may inhibit prostaglandin production (Backon, 1989). High ß-endorphin may then prevent cervical ripening.

The brain's right of veto

Stress hormones influence behaviour aimed at modifying the environment. If high stress hormones can delay the onset of labour then the mother is given the chance to modify or choose the environment in which she gives birth. If the mother's environment is causing her stress, her hypothalamus may carry on producing ACT hormone and ß-endorphin on top of progesterone-induced ACT hormone and ß-endorphin. These hormones will then continue to lock her uterus and her cervix into holding on to her child, even when the child has signalled its willingness to be born. When the mother is no longer stressed, that is, when her physical environment matches bodily needs better, then labour can start. Pregnancy is then, I think, epitomised by high natural maternal stress levels, and the onset of labour may well be release from pregnancy-induced stress hormone secretion.

The hormonal evidence

My theory implies that a woman should have low ACT hormone levels and thus low cortisol levels to go into labour normally. Horses and seals have both been found to be able to delay labour until circumstances are favourable (Racey, 1981). Low cortisol levels have been found in women giving birth spontaneously at term. Kauppila and Tuimala (1974) found a positive correlation between length of labour, and ACT hormone and cortisol at the start of an induced labour. Induction of labour for postmaturity is common in clinical practice, although whether or not postmaturity is more common in women who are afraid of childbirth itself is not known. Perhaps the degree of fear may make a difference. If a mother is absolutely terrified, she may go into premature labour, but if only mildly fearful she may go past her expected date of confinement.

There are very many ways in which this hypothesis may be tested, and some people may say that I should wait until more research has been done in order to put it to the test. But I feel that there is already enough biochemical and hormonal evidence to present the case. The hypothesis needs to be aired, and mothers and midwives need to be aware of possible connections between stress, prematurity and the onset of labour. It will take years for research into this theory to be done, but meanwhile action taken to reduce stress in late pregnancy may save very many babies from prematurity and many women from induction of labour for stress-induced postmaturity.

The right environment for labour?

Why should a stress-free environment for birth be so significant for the onset of labour in horses and seals – and humans? Again the laws of natural selection provide the answer. Labouring in a stress-free environment has survival value for mother and child. Natural selection would not put the life of the foetus at risk through postmaturity unless there was a selective advantage to the child of being born in a favourable environment.

This is fairly easy to grasp for animals. Offspring born to mothers in safe places away from predators would be more likely to survive than those born in dangerous situations. But I suggest that it was the *place of labour* for the mother as well as place of birth for the child that was important in evolution. I am convinced that labour proceeds more smoothly if the mother is spared unnecessary stress. High levels of stress hormones interfere with the process of labour itself, particularly in the early stages. The mother survived childbirth to bear more children if she chose to labour in a safe place, and throughout the animal world, that place is the nest.

Since both mother and foetus have a vested interest in surviving childbirth, they should co-ordinate their efforts to ensure that the time is right for both. The time is right for the foetus when it is ready to breathe for itself; and the time is right for the mother when she is physically and mentally prepared for labour. There is no conflict of interest between mother and child – each wants the other to come through the process unscathed and prepared for the new life ahead.

The million dollar question is of course, what constitutes a safe place? For animals we have no trouble in stating that the safest place is the nest, but for humans the politics of the maternity services revolve precisely round this very question. Most people maintain that hospital is the safest place for mother and child in labour while a few, myself included are convinced that home birth is just as safe if not safer, and certainly less painful and more enjoyable.

Who is right or, indeed, are both right? Should pregnant women have more choice in childbirth? If an individual's *perception* of safety is important, then some women will feel safer in hospital and some safer at home. We can even distinguish between the two groups physically by measuring blood pressure and pulse rate in hospital antenatal clinics. Women with raised blood pressure and pulse rate over rates measured at home or in a GP clinic should be advised that it may be safer for them to deliver at home or in a GP unit.

As recently as 1984, when only 1% of mothers had a home birth, a surprising number of women (16%) felt that women should have the option of home birth if they wanted it (Morgan *et al*, 1984). Ninety-two percent of women who had a home birth following a hospital confinement preferred the home birth (O'Brien, 1975). Dutch statistics show a perinatal death rate of 18 per thousand for deliveries in consultant units in the presence of a doctor and a death rate of just one in a thousand for babies born at home in the presence of just a midwife (Tew, 1990).

The House of Commons committee chaired by Nicholas Winterton MP came out in favour of home birth (HMSO, 1992) and the National Perinatal Epidemiology Unit has similarly questioned the advantages of hospital birth (*Where to be Born? The debate and the evidence*, Campbell and Macfarlane, 1987). The increased statistical danger of hospital birth has been put very strongly by Marjorie Tew (*Safer Childbirth?* 1990) who suggested that there could be a hidden advantage of home birth. I suggest the hidden advantage to be the stress free environment of home.

But authors, politicians and statisticians should not have the last word – the woman herself should decide for herself. She should labour where she feels safest which may be in a consultant unit, a GP unit or at home as she thinks fit. And her decision should be founded on scientific facts rather than medical fictions.

4 The Womb

"This fortress built by Nature for herself against infection... "
Shakespeare, Richard II

Anatomy and Function of the Uterus

No one can hope to understand the process of normal childbirth without understanding how the uterus works. The standard medical approach to uterine function is to assume that maternal behaviour has very little to do with childbirth but in fact the opposite is the case. As with other organs such as the heart, the uterus is very much influenced by the mental processes of the woman owning it; the psychology of uterine function is as important as the physiology. However, for the moment, I will consider the function of the uterus in isolation and forget that it is an integral part of an intelligent human being whose behaviour is affected by a multitude of psychological factors.

Pregnancy and childbirth depend on the fundamental biological requirement for a uterus first to contain a foetus for nine months and then to contract and expel its contents at term. The well established medical discipline of the science of childbirth deals almost exclusively with the physical action of the uterus. Biochemists are interested in what makes it contract and what makes it relax, and endocrinologists are interested in control of this process by the pituitary gland and hypothalamus. Despite the interest from neuroendocrinologists, the role of emotions seems to be largely ignored. I will start to put some of the hormones of pregnancy and labour into the context of childbirth in the following chapter but, for the moment, will describe the functions and mechanics of the uterus because it is impossible to understand how hormones can act upon it without knowing its anatomy and physiology.

Childbirth is the most complex process in the mammalian life cycle, involving enormous changes to the bodies of both mother and child in a very short space of time. Comparable changes to the body at puberty and on becoming pregnant take place relatively slowly over months or years, but childbirth happens within the space of a few hours. The mother is suddenly no longer pregnant; the child is suddenly separated from her and obtains his oxygen from the air instead of his mother's blood. Indeed, for the first time in his life, theoretically, the child is able to do without his mother. For the child there is a sudden transition from total bodily dependence to total bodily independence; for the mother there is the sudden relief from the demands of a parasite that has been invading her body for the last nine months or so, and a sudden transition into the very different demands of motherhood. Such radical changes happening in so short a time demand very drastic, purposeful action by the mother's body. For the process to be completed safely for mother and child the mechanism must be finely tuned to optimise the chance of success.

Natural selection has made subtle changes to the action of the uterus over millions of years; changing the organ itself, selecting new hormones to act on it, and changing its responsiveness to pre-existing hormones.

The uterus – a dual purpose organ

The uterus is required to fulfil two distinct, diametrically opposed biological functions: to provide a safe environment for a growing foetus for nine months, and to expel its contents at the end of that time safely and efficiently. It is amazing how well one organ can perform these two conflicting functions; during pregnancy the uterus is already preparing to rid itself of its burden while at the same time it is jealously protecting the foetus from the outside world. For nine months the mother's body sustains and nurtures the foetus as if it were part of herself but, at term, the foetus is at last recognised as a foreign body, and treated accordingly – expelled. The uterus must provide access to nutrients from the mother for the growing foetus and then cut off the supply abruptly, to prevent haemorrhage after the birth. It has to screen the foetus from the outside world for nine months and then it must suddenly withdraw this protection and provide a doorway to the outside world via the cervix. It has to expand with the growing foetus and then revert to its previous size and prepare for the next baby. The uterus is one of the most complex organs in the body; it is the largest and, arguably, the most powerful muscle. It undergoes fundamental changes throughout the menstrual cycle, pregnancy and labour. It is influenced by a wider variety of hormones than any other organ.

Because of its importance in reproduction, natural selection allowed the female no voluntary control over the workings of her own uterus; a woman can usually choose to delay urination and defecation but she cannot choose a convenient time for ovulation, menstruation or labour; her hormones choose those times for her. The advent of the Pill was perhaps the first time in the history of the world that the power of natural selection was curtailed by giving man real power over reproduction.

Involuntary elastic muscle

The womb is an elastic bag with elastic memory. Like any other sort of elastic, if it is stretched it will spring back into shape. It will actually become more elastic at the place where it is stretched. Elastic muscle is called smooth, involuntary, or visceral muscle by the anatomists. When the layman thinks of muscle he thinks of biceps and triceps, weightlifting and physical strength. Elastic muscle, particularly uterine muscle, is just as strong but it is controlled in a different way. Biceps and triceps are skeletal muscle and we can control skeletal muscle by acts of will. We decide to walk and instinctively activate the relevant muscles for walking. But we cannot decide for ourselves when to make elastic muscle work. Uterine muscle is involuntary, and is under the dual control of the autonomic nervous system (that part of the nervous system which the brain leaves largely to organise itself) and the hormonal system. Elastic muscle is worked by hormonal, biochemical and electrical innate reflexes. It is found in the hollow organs of the body, the heart, blood vessels, digestive tract and the uterus. The two types of muscle work in different ways. Skeletal muscle is like a spring that needs energy to be made smaller (contract) and smooth muscle, like elastic, needs energy to resist contracting. Uterine muscle contracts as a response to being stretched. It has the further unique quality of becoming even smaller than its original size – as if stretching household elastic could actually shorten the original length.

The powers of the hormonal forces that prevent the pregnant, and therefore stretched, uterus from resisting its innate tendency to contract are enormous. It is almost easier to understand how the uterus contracts in labour than to understand how it resists contracting in pregnancy. The foetus in its own bag of amniotic fluid is continually stretching the uterus in pregnancy and, as both foetus and uterus grow, more and more pressure is exerted on the weakest part of the elastic muscular bag, the cervix, the outlet for the baby. If household elastic were continuously stretched for months at a time it would lose its elasticity but uterine muscle actually gains elasticity. It has returned to its previous size by a fortnight or so after birth.

The hormones of pregnancy, particularly progesterone and ß-endorphin, act as a brake on uterine activity. The first stage of labour proceeds as the hormonal brakes are gradually taken away and only during the second stage does the uterus use its full expulsive powers.

Since we cannot make smooth muscle work by an act of will, the only way of influencing it is to use indirect, psychological means – changing our state of mind and thus altering the secretion of stress hormones.

Contractions

Unlike voluntary muscle which is relaxed unless we instruct it to act, involuntary muscle contracts spontaneously all the time. Involuntary muscle is responsible for the subconscious innate reflex workings of the body: it supports life-maintaining functions: the heart pumps the blood around the body, the blood vessels direct the blood to the right places, the gut digests food, the lungs take in oxygen. And the uterus carries life forward to the next generation. These automatic functions are too important to leave to the whims of the individual, and the subconscious retains control of them.

Skeletal muscle contracts only when it receives nervous impulses, but smooth muscle twitches spontaneously in a test tube in the absence of any nervous input. Uterine muscle contracts spontaneously all the time, whether or not a woman is pregnant, and nervous and hormonal input enhances, inhibits or co-ordinates contractions. Uterine muscle contracts in two ways, conveniently labelled A and B. A contractions are spontaneous contractions that maintain muscle tone. Any muscle that is not used wastes away and, at least until the menopause, uterine muscle is constantly preparing for the next labour. A contractions are irregular and unco-ordinated. B contractions are the Braxton Hicks contractions of late pregnancy and labour; they enable the uterus to act as a whole rather than as a collection of individual muscle fibres. Braxton Hicks contractions are the regular, co-ordinated contractions that will lead eventually to the expulsion of the foetus. Throughout pregnancy uterine muscle is being prepared for the co-ordinated **B** contractions of labour.

Specialised muscle

Uterine muscle has the capacity for great expansion. The enormous increase in the size of the uterus throughout pregnancy is achieved through a tenfold increase in cell size and a fifteenfold increase in cell length rather than an increase in the actual number of cells. Muscle cells have grown to ten times their original size by the twentieth week of pregnancy. After that time the muscle stretches more and more to accommodate the growing foetus. Given that uterine muscle contracts as a reflex response to being stretched, the disparity between the increase in size (x 10) and the increase in length (x 15) gives some idea of the strength of the hormonal forces acting on the muscle during the second half of pregnancy. Ever more powerful hormonal input is needed to resist the innate tendency to contract. Maternal blood ß-endorphin levels rise again in the third trimester of pregnancy (Hoffman *et al*, 1984).

The bag of muscle is composed of three (or even four, according to one authority, Elstein and Chantler, 1990) separate sets of muscle: longitudinal muscle running up and over the uterus; latitudinal muscle; and in between these two layers, diagonal muscle fibres spiralling round the uterus in opposite directions. If three sets of fibres have evolved one would expect them to perform different functions, and this seems to be the case. The longitudinal muscle is the most powerful and has the task of dilating the cervix, opening the womb's door, in the first stage of labour, and pushing the foetus down the birth canal in the second stage. The latitudinal muscle is mainly responsible for keeping the cervix shut during pregnancy. The spiralling muscle steers the presenting part of the foetus towards the cervix.

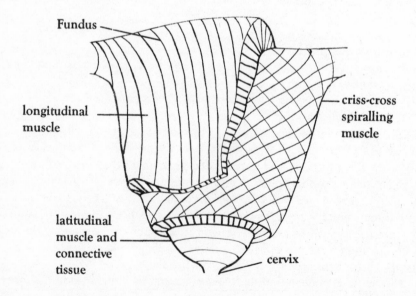

13: Muscle layers in the uterus

The Womb's a Balloon

The uterus can be compared to a balloon – but unlike a normal party balloon it actually grows to ten times its original size, in the first twenty weeks.

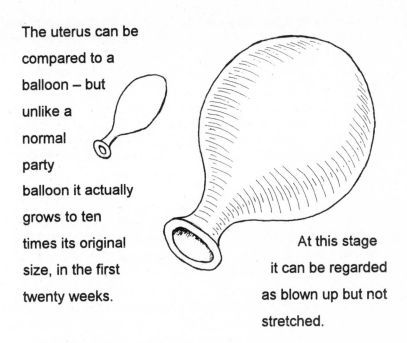

At this stage it can be regarded as blown up but not stretched.

In the second twenty weeks it stretches, so that at term it is half as large again, or fifteen times larger than at the start.

Unlike the party balloon it has no knot. The door is shut by hormones.

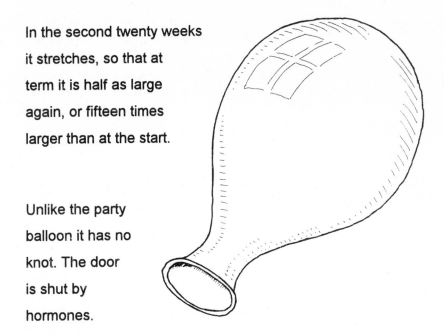

The expulsive muscle at the top of the uterus, the fundus, is mainly longitudinal muscle. The lower end of the uterus is composed of only 10% muscle which is mainly latitudinal muscle, the rest of the tissue being a network of non-muscular (connective) tissue and held together tightly with hormone bonds during pregnancy. The cervix is the foetus' gateway to the outside world and remains tightly shut until hormonal bonds are loosened and the gate is pulled up out of the way by the longitudinal muscle fibres of the uterus.

Thus, during labour, the longitudinal muscle contracts while the latitudinal muscle is stretched to its limits to open the cervix. There seems to be very little information about qualitative differences between the three uterine muscle types, some researchers state that they experiment on fundal strips, that is mainly longitudinal muscle, but more often the type of muscle is not stated, merely labelled as uterine strip. This may be because it is difficult to distinguish between the different muscle layers by eye. One group of researchers in Japan have found significant differences between longitudinal and latitudinal muscle in pigs regarding both biochemistry and function which reflect the opposing role of these two types of muscle in pregnancy and labour (Taneike *et al*, 1991).

Blood supply
The uterus is supplied with blood from two sources, from the uterine arteries at the lower end and the ovarian arteries at the top. Thus it receives hormonal input both from blood coming directly from the ovaries, and also from blood coming from the general circulation. The hormonal content of blood from different sources will be different. Blood coming from the ovaries will contain a greater proportion of hormones secreted by the ovaries than blood in the general circulation. The top of the uterus, the fundus, being near to the ovaries, receives most of its blood from the ovarian arteries. Blood from the two sources mingles about half way down the uterus. Thus the fundal expulsive muscle will be mainly fed by blood containing ovarian hormones and latitudinal muscle at the lower end, near the cervix, will fed by blood that has bypassed the ovaries.

The network of blood vessels can also carry hormones released from one part of the uterus to another part. Prostaglandins are local hormones produced by ordinary cells which are not specialised for mass hormone production as are, for example the ovaries or adrenal glands. They are produced locally and have effects in cells near the source cell. A prostaglandin vaginal pessary given to induce labour will exert its effects locally, that is at the cervical end of the uterus.

Nerve supply to the uterus
The nerve supply *to* the uterus is via the parasympathetic nervous system – that part of the nervous system which provides automatic reflex control of the body as opposed to voluntary control. On the other hand, nerves *from* the uterus provide sensory input to the sympathetic nervous system – that part of the

nervous system of which we are more aware. If nervous supply to the uterus is cut off (in women who have a damaged spinal cord, or having epidural block pain relief in labour) the uterus works more effectively during the first stage of labour. This implies that nerves play more of a negative role in labour than a positive one. Medical students are taught that parasympathetic nerves have "little importance in uterine activity" (Llewellyn-Jones, 1990) but, arguing from evolution, I have to maintain that these nerves must serve a useful purpose or they would not exist at all. Moreover, uterine sympathetic nerves become more sensitive in pregnancy, not less sensitive. This implies an important physiological role for nervous input during labour. The ability of the brain to perceive pain must have survival value for both mother and child. One biological role of pain is to promote instinctive pain-avoidance behaviour in order to remove the underlying cause of the pain. If the underlying cause is removed labour will proceed more efficiently. If pain is not felt then pain-avoidance behaviour will not take place.

Nerve supply below the uterus
The nerves of the pelvis, the diaphragm and abdomen are part of the sympathetic nervous system which is under voluntary control and, unlike uterine nerves, these nerves have a positive role to play in labour. During the second stage of labour the mother's instincts are called upon; she becomes a voluntary partner with her involuntary uterus for the hardest work of labour, pushing the foetus out into the world. The voluntary skeletal muscles of the diaphragm, pelvis and abdomen are used by the mother to assist the fundal uterine muscle to expel the foetus. Nervous information from these parts is acted on instinctively and consciously instead of by reflex action, for example we are able to tighten anal muscles at will and to relax them when necessary to expel waste products. Animal scientists investigating birth in rabbits found, somewhat to their surprise, that nervous signals from these parts at birth closely resembled nervous signals at defecation. To many mothers this information would come as no surprise at all.

Epidural anaesthesia cuts out nervous signals from the vagina and perineum, removing the urge to push at the same time as blocking pain. In these circumstances the mother must rely on being told when to push; or she must wait for the effects of an epidural block to wear off, or the baby is delivered by forceps.

Simultaneous Opposing Role of the Uterus During Labour

During labour the uterus switches from being a protective cocoon for the foetus to being a powerful expulsive organ. Labour may take place in a relatively short space of time but the foetus still needs to be protected from the violent forces of labour. Its oxygen lifeline must not be compromised.

The uterus retains its protective role towards the foetus throughout the first two stages of labour in one site – at the placenta. Uterine muscle at the placental site remains resistant to hormones promoting contractions. During labour the uterus must continue to provide a good blood supply to the foetus and to protect the vulnerable placental site from the powerful expulsive contractions of the second stage of labour which might tear the placenta from the uterus and deprive the foetus of oxygen. Abruptio placenta is the medical term describing this separation. It endangers the life of the foetus by reducing the oxygen supply.

During labour, therefore, the uterus performs its two opposing functions at one and the same time. The placental site continues to resist hormonal instructions for contractions, while the rest of the uterus performs the expulsive contractions of labour. This split in function is brought about by action of placental hormones on the part of the uterus that is touching the placenta.

The placenta is the site of progesterone and ß-endorphin production and, because progesterone is a small steroid hormone, it can filter through cell membranes as well as entering the blood stream for diffusion. The placental site, being closer to the site of production, will receive more progesterone than the rest of the uterus. From the very beginning of placental hormone production the placental site is prepared for the need to resist hormonal instructions to contract in labour.

Uterine muscle cells at the placental site grow bigger than cells elsewhere. Surgeons performing caesarean sections noticed that they could predict the placental site by a bulge seen from outside the uterus before they cut into uterine muscle. This bulge acts as a cushion to prevent placental uterine muscle stretching, and therefore contracting, during the first two stages of labour. Once the baby is born the placenta separates, and the placental site can also contract for the third stage of labour. I suspect that foetal hormones also have a role to play in maintaining the resistance of the placental site to contractions in the first and second stages of labour. Once the cord is cut foetal blood no longer reaches the placental site and the placental site starts to lose its resistance to contractions.

When the placenta is situated at the top of the uterus, where the muscle is thickest and most powerful (in about 3% of pregnancies, although numerous textbooks show this placental site as the normal position), labour tends to be longer since some of the most powerful muscle is prevented from contracting. Also these women have a higher incidence of retained placenta and post-partum haemorrhage, suggesting a different hormonal response of fundal muscle. Placental site can be detected by ultrasound so these problems can be predicted before labour starts. Women can be warned to expect a longer than average labour. This is still no reason for enforced hospital birth; it is rather a contraindication since hospital staff may find it almost impossible to resist intervening in prolonged labour. Flying squads or ambulances can be ready with matched blood in case the mother haemorrhages. In hospital, birth attendants will know to allow women longer at each stage of labour and be less rigid about accelerating labour and performing caesarean sections for uterine inertia.

Direction of Labour by the Uterus and the Foetus

Standard medical opinion seems to suggest that contractions always spread from the fallopian tubes outwards. This is certainly the case in lower mammals but in humans, according to some authorities, the pacemaker, or centre of propagating contractions varies (Csapo, 1966). I suggest that this change took place in evolution with the appearance of the unicornate uterus and the change from the cylindrical position of the foetus to the oval foetal position of primates. This suggests a far more important role for uterine muscle in humans than simply providing power for expulsion.

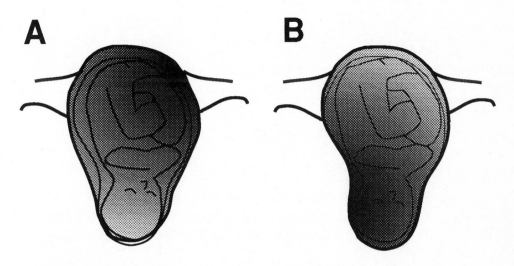

15: Spread of contractions.
A – classic theory
B – contraction initiated by foetal pressure

If the centre of propagating contractions varies according to the degree of stretch imparted by the foetus, then the uterus can act purposefully to fold the foetus into the oval position ready for birth in prelabour, and to guide the presenting part (usually the head) to the uterine outlet during the first stage of labour.

The criss-cross elastic of a trampoline is designed to direct the trampolinist back into the centre of the trampoline, and the criss-cross spiralling uterine muscle is designed to steer the foetus into the centre of the uterus. During labour, however, the latitudinal muscle does not respond to stretch by contracting, which implies that the spiralling muscle can steer the foetus downwards. The relaxation of the latitudinal muscle changes the mechanical dynamics of the uterus.

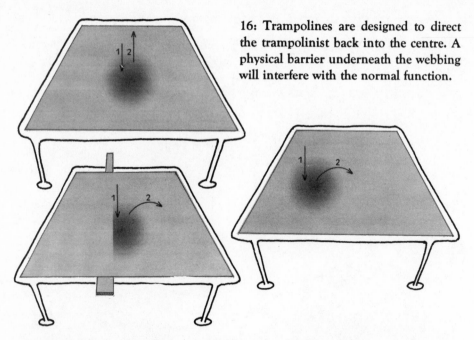

16: Trampolines are designed to direct the trampolinist back into the centre. A physical barrier underneath the webbing will interfere with the normal function.

During the first stage of labour, therefore, the foetus and the uterus dance an intricate *pas de deux* which directs the foetus towards the cervix to be ideally placed for the second stage of labour, the passage of the foetus through the cervix and down the vagina to the outside world.

The implication for labour is that the mother should be allowed freedom of movement in order to give full rein to these directed contractions. I suggest that painful contractions occur when the uterus is prevented from working as it should. If the mother is confined to one position and the foetus gets into an awkward position, uterine muscle may be prevented from stretching by forces outside the uterus and so contractions may slow down or lose their intensity, prolonging labour and exhausting the mother. Returning to the analogy of the trampoline, the trampoline will be prevented from working properly if a pole is

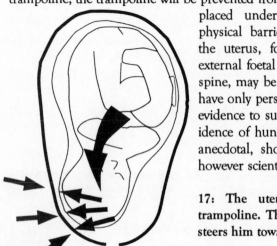

placed under the elastic webbing. Any physical barrier inhibiting the elasticity of the uterus, for example the girdle of an external foetal monitor or the mother's own spine, may be similarly counterproductive. I have only personal experience and anecdotal evidence to support this opinion but the evidence of hundreds of women, even if only anecdotal, should not be ignored entirely, however scientific we would wish to remain.

17: The uterus is like a pear shaped trampoline. The pressure of the baby's head steers him towards the outlet

Hydraulics

If the waters remain unbroken throughout the first stage of labour then the effect of a cushion of amniotic fluid between the baby and the uterus will be to spread the foetal force more evenly. If the waters are broken then the presenting part will exert a larger effect over a smaller area and thus lead to the more violent first stage contractions that follow artificial rupture of the membranes (ARM) in early labour.

Of course, for some women, labour appears to start with rupture of the membranes, but for these women labour is usually already well established without the mother being aware of the fact. Although contractions will necessarily become more powerful than they were before the waters broke, there will less of a jump between the weak contractions of late pregnancy and the powerful contractions that come late in the first stage of labour. It was probably a particularly powerful contraction that broke the waters in the first place.

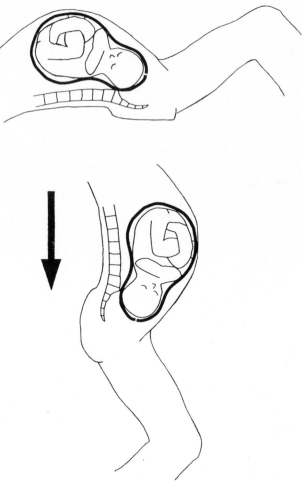

18: Imagine the effect of gravity on labour in these two women

Freedom of movement

Man has a very finely developed sense of balance, dating from the time he swung from branch to branch in the antediluvian forests, and further developed when he started to walk and stand upright. This sense of knowing one's position in space (termed proprioception by psychologists) depends on a highly developed network of nerves and reflex adjustments. Although no one seems to have done any research into instinctive changes of maternal position during labour, the biological mechanism for instinctive position changing to maintain balance is already in existence and I see no reason why labouring women should not be able to co-ordinate bodily position with site of contractions.

Freedom of movement is a cornerstone of instinctive childbirth. Immobility is a recipe for obstetric disaster, as will become readily apparent in later chapters.

Psychology of Uterine Function

There can be little doubt that the first stage of labour is under automatic subconscious control. All the indications seem to suggest that the uterus works best in the first stage of labour when left to its own devices. Where there is any input from the sympathetic nervous system to the uterus, it inhibits rather than promotes labour. The first stage of labour seems to me to be a normal bodily process under the control of the subconscious. Conscious interference in the natural process takes place only when the brain exercises its right of veto and slows down contractions. The brain exercises this right when something is wrong and action is required of the mother. Pain is a signal to the mother that something is wrong and that something should be done.

Some women go through the first stage of labour without even knowing that they are in labour. They do not feel any pain in the first stage because their brain sees no need to tell them to change either their position or their surroundings. Not all women caught short and having their babies in cars or ambulances by the roadside have wilfully delayed their journey to hospital; on the contrary, labour was going so well that the brain saw no need to tell the mother that she was in labour. It is not until the second stage that the body needs much help from the mother.

Efficient uterine function depends on nervous, hormonal and biochemical messages being passed to and fro between the uterus and the brain via the nervous system and the hormonal system. Any disruption of these messages is likely to reduce efficiency in childbearing. My argument for returning control of labour to women themselves rests on the theory that medical control of childbirth disrupts biochemical messages between uterus and brain and is bound to lead to pain and danger through upsetting natural checks and balances evolved over millions of years of natural selection. It goes without saying that a woman feels most in control when on her own ground, at home, and least in control in hospital, where control is taken out of her hands.

100

THE ART
OF
CHILDBIRTH

5   Labour

"And all shall be well, and all shall be well, and all manner of things shall be well."

Julian of Norwich

For sixty years or more scientists have been suspending strips of animal and human uterus in various liquids in test tubes, stretching it, adding hormones, adding chemicals, measuring contractions, analysing changes, and generally trying to find out what makes uterine muscle work and what stops it working. Laboratory animals and human subjects have been injected with various substances in various parts of the uterus, the placenta, the amniotic fluid and the foetus; and in various parts of the brain in an effort to unravel the mystery of labour. Levels of hormones in foetal and maternal blood have been extensively studied by endocrinologists and obstetricians in attempts to find predictors of foetal distress.

Unfortunately there seems to have been little communication between the endocrinologists, biochemists and the medical establishment. Where scientists have discovered a compound that acts on the uterus, obstetricians have seized upon it to add to their battery of drugs for managing labour, but they have not seen beyond "therapeutic" uses. They have missed the opportunities to increase their understanding of normal labour. One example of this is the contraction-stopping action of adrenaline. Adrenaline was found to stop contractions in the 1920s, and obstetricians experimented with it in an attempt to prevent premature labour. But they did not see the implication that labouring women should be freed from unnecessary stress.

The various groups of scientists seem to be very wary of each other, each talking of the other in disparaging terms as if they were enemies instead of partners in solving the mysteries of labour. The obstetricians despised the scientists for their lack of clinical experience, and the biochemists and endocrinologists despised the doctors for their limited knowledge of pure science. One biochemist described the active management of labour (oxytocin infusion to speed up labour) as *pharmacological accouchment forcé* and was disparaged by an obstetrician at a symposium as being an advocate of *hopeful procrastination* (Csapo, 1961). Feelings on intervention in labour run as high among the scientists as in the women they serve. None of the groups seems to have considered the psychological implications of the pure research at all. If they have, they have not deemed it important enough to act on the increased knowledge. The scientists have completely ignored the mother herself and her mind. This is why obstetrics is the least scientifically based medical specialty. But stress hormones unlock the mysteries of labour itself.

Labour is controlled by hormones. Each hormone has a specific job to do and hormone secretion is regulated by the brain. The hormonal control of labour is very complex and difficult to understand but it has certain similarities with driving a car.

The mother's brain is the driver and her uterus is the engine. The baby is his mother's eyes in that his position inside her determines which way to turn the steering wheel. The three pedals control hormones. The clutch represents oestrogen, the foot brake represents adrenaline and the accelerator represents oxytocin. A car will come to a stop in three ways: by depressing the clutch and disengaging the engine, by stopping petrol supplies reaching the engine and by using the foot brake. In pregnancy and labour these functions are performed by stress hormones. As well as maintaining pregnancy, stress hormones control labour by regulating the power of the uterine engine.

The role of a birth attendant should be like that of a driving instructor rather than a back-seat driver. Education and encouragement are more helpful than grabbing the steering wheel and slamming on the dual control foot brake whenever the smallest mistake is made. A learner continually subjected to panic reactions by the instructor will lose self-confidence and may give up altogether. The better the driving instructor, the less likely learners are to crash and need the emergency services.

If the driver relies too much on the advice of a back-seat driver, particularly one who has never driven before but has learnt all he knows through watching other people drive cars, she is more likely to have an accident. If she lets the back-seat driver completely control her labour she is asking for trouble.

The Controls

The action of the three pedals of a car has to be synchronised for it to be driven smoothly and safely. ß-endorphin is the natural regulator of labour hormones. During pregnancy and the first stage of labour it prevents the engine from becoming fully engaged by "jamming" oestrogen receptors at the hypothalamus, and at the uterus itself. During the second stage of labour it regulates oxytocin secretion.

The handbrake

The connective tissue bonds holding the cervix tightly closed during pregnancy can be thought of as the handbrake. For a few women the handbrake is not strong enough to keep the cervix tightly locked and the pregnancy miscarries – this is a problem caused mainly by bipedalism – in quadrupeds the physical pressure exerted by the foetus will not be applied to the cervix but elsewhere in the uterus. An artificial handbrake of stitches can be applied to solve this problem; the stitches are removed when pregnancy has reached term.

Labour can start only when the handbrake is taken off as the cervix is ripened by prostaglandins. Sometimes the handbrake is taken off too soon, a different biological role for prostaglandins is to fight infection and there is a definite link between premature delivery and pelvic infection. The cervix must be softened and pliable before labour can start in earnest. Once it is softened then labour can start.

The clutch

In a car the function of the clutch is to enable the power of an engine to be transmitted to the driving wheels; oestrogen wires up the uterus for co-ordinated contractions thus engaging the uterine engine. ß-endorphin stops the clutch from being raised.

The foot brake

The foot brake is available for unforeseen emergencies and using the foot brake means taking one's foot off the accelerator. Adrenaline is the foot brake.

The accelerator

This pedal is used to increase petrol supplies to the engine enabling it to work harder. Oxytocin controls the fuel supply to the uterus. Ideally, the speed of the car can be controlled by using the accelerator and clutch to match engine speed and gears to road conditions. ß-endorphin stops the accelerator from being pressed.

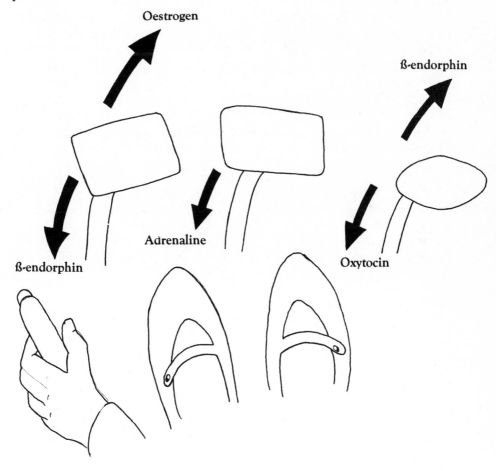

19: Adrenaline is the foot brake while ß-endorphin disengages the engine and reduces petrol supply.

Pregnancy

Since uterine muscle is smooth muscle that is always active unless it is switched off, we can compare it to a car engine that is running, though not necessarily driving the wheels. Most of the time, in non-pregnant women, the uterus is idling in neutral – it has small bursts of activity at ovulation, at sexual intercourse, and at menstruation but, apart from women unlucky enough to suffer from period pains, these contractions usually remain below the threshold of consciousness.

On becoming pregnant there is a fundamental change to the state of the uterus – it remains in neutral but at the same time gradually prepares itself for the hard work of driving the muscle that will push the baby out. Progesterone and oestrogen put it into gear while at the same time progesterone and ß-endorphin depress the clutch, disengaging the engine.

Prelabour

Progesterone and ß-endorphin stop co-ordinated contractions. Like a depressed clutch, they prevent the transfer of power from the engine to the driving wheels. ß-endorphin competes with oestrogen in wiring up the uterus – engaging the engine. A car will not move itself with the clutch completely depressed; the clutch has to be engaged to transmit power from the engine to the driving wheels.

The action of the clutch can be varied: we can slip the clutch to move slowly in traffic jams. The degree of depression of the clutch determines the amount of power that is transmitted to the engine. In pregnancy the doses of clutch depression hormones, progesterone and ß-endorphin, are large enough to prevent any power being transmitted at all. Towards term the hormonal clutch pedal is raised slightly from time to time. Braxton Hicks contractions, the practice labour contractions, occur. But because the uterus has not yet been wired up for labour by oestrogen, these contractions are not strong enough to engage the full power of the uterus, and labour does not start. These contractions are like testing the clutch in an unfamiliar car to see where the biting point is before starting to move off in earnest.

Onset of labour

A ripe cervix is one precondition for labour to start – the hormonal handbrake must be taken off before labour can proceed normally. However, prelabour gradually merges into labour proper, the handbrake is gradually taken off and contractions gradually cross the threshold into consciousness. (This is like a hill start in a car.) Other signs that women are taught to look for are a *show*, the discharge of a mucous plug from the vagina, or spontaneous rupture of the membranes, although labour does not always start after either of these events.

Since the onset of labour is insidious, the practical definition of the onset of labour is somewhat arbitrary. The medical definition of the onset of labour used to be regular *painful* contractions. Nowadays the word painful is excluded from the definition, which is an advance, but professionals prefer to decide for themselves whether a woman is in labour or not, by using such measures as degree of cervical dilatation. But even cervical dilatation is not enough to be certain that labour has started – women can have the cervix open up to 4 cm without being in active labour. Doctors would rather not take a woman's word for it that she has regular contractions. They cover themselves for the fact that many women come to hospital because regular contractions have started only to find that contractions stop on arrival at hospital. This could be better described as arrested labour rather than labelled a false alarm and is in itself a powerful argument for the role of stress hormones in regulating labour.

I think the confusion surrounding the onset of labour lies in when the mother *becomes conscious* that she is in labour; when she realises that her uterus is starting to behave differently. Some women fail to know that they are in labour at all until the second stage has started. They may have a sudden urge to defecate only to discover that their baby is just about to be born. For them the first stage of labour was fully subconscious. I believe that this is how it used to be when the world was young and we still lacked the ability to talk to each other and to discover from each other what signalled a new baby's arrival. Cats do not stray far from home when labour is imminent and indeed some women feel unusually lethargic the day before labour, while others may become very energetic – nest-building activity preparing for the new baby. Both staying at home and nest-building activity reduce stress hormone secretion and help to remove the block on the uterus.

The conscious onset of labour may be preceded by unusual bodily activity. A woman who has suffered from constipation during pregnancy may suddenly have loose stools again. This is a sign of the withdrawal of the progesterone-induced ß-endorphin block on the bowel, a side effect of the ß-endorphin block on the uterus. Although it still may be some hours before uterine contractions cross the threshold into consciousness, the first stage of labour has already started. Looser bowels movements often precede and accompany menstruation, another time when a ß-endorphin block on the uterus and bowel is removed.

The Three Stages of Labour

The three stages of labour divide neatly into three physical and hormonal phases. The hormones secreted in each of the three phases reflect both the physical progress of labour and the mental state of the mother. The mother's psychological state must be right and hormones correctly balanced for each stage for labour to proceed smoothly and safely.

The First Stage

Labour starts in earnest when hormones promoting contractions start to predominate over hormones inhibiting contractions. In the car analogy the car starts to move just after the clutch biting point is reached and the handbrake is taken off so that the engine is allowed to drive the wheels. The whole of the first stage of labour is like gradually taking one's foot off the hormonal clutch of the uterus and gradually releasing the handbrake. Slowly the whole of the uterine engine becomes engaged and able to act as a single unit – except at the placental site where the ß-endorphin block is maintained and even strengthened by increased doses of ß-endorphin from the baby's blood and CRF in addition to, or perhaps instead of, progesterone.

The first stage is the removal of the progesterone and ß-endorphin block on uterine smooth muscle – a gradual removing of clutch depression hormone which allows more and more of the uterus to be wired up with oestrogen. As oestrogen replaces ß-endorphin at the uterus, more and more muscle is brought into action and linked together electrically to allow contractions to spread. The same blood level of oxytocin that was present at the end of pregnancy has an increasingly greater effect. Receiving stations for oxytocin become more numerous throughout the first stage of labour only to fall back again once the whole of the available uterine engine is wired up. More and more muscle becomes hormonally primed to respond to oxytocin.

The car is being manoeuvred out of its garage and the doors are gradually opening automatically – the cervix dilates. As longitudinal muscle contracts, latitudinal muscle at the cervix relaxes and a gateway to the outside world is made. The uterus itself is becoming part of the birth canal and the baby slowly edges into the pelvis.

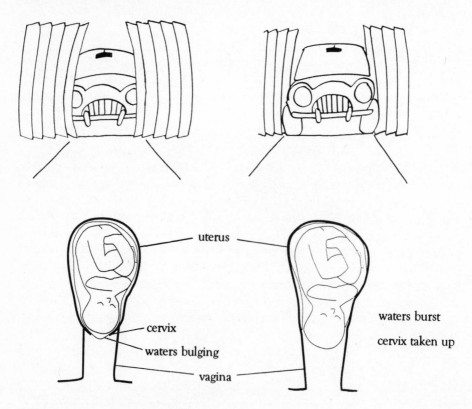

20: The start of the journey proper

During this stage the baby is being manoeuvred into the best position for the birth itself. The passenger, the baby, is telling the mother's uterus which way to steer by physical pressure against different parts of it – "Left hand down a bit... Right hand down a bit... Keep going." The pressure of the baby himself decides where the centre of each contraction will be in the first stage. Every so often the mother fails to respond to one of these pressure instructions, hits an obstacle and experiences pain. She slows down to recover her breath and then starts again. If she does not listen to his instructions at all then the process of getting out of the garage will be haphazard, slow and painful. The pain tells her that she is not listening to the instructions. Being forced to stay in the same position throughout labour is a bit like having the steering wheel locked when trying to manoeuvre a car. If the mother is confined to bed or physically constrained she may be physically unable to respond to instinctive cues for pain-avoidance behaviour. Although the uterus is doing all the real work automatically, the mother must respond to instructions from her body to give it ideal working conditions.

First stage contractions

The first stage of labour emerges from the same hormonal conditions that prevailed in late pregnancy. Braxton Hicks contractions just happened during the prelabour days, they were controlled subconsciously and automatically then, and still are during labour. The only difference is that now the mother becomes aware of them. For some women contractions do not cross the threshold into consciousness until very late in labour. This means that all is going well. Most of the lay birth books state that when a baby comes too soon to allow time for transfer to hospital then it usually means that the birth will be easy.

Contractions cannot become strong enough to convert a quiescent uterus into an efficiently labouring uterus if stress hormone secretion is too high. It follows that stress hormone secretion should remain as low as possible throughout the first stage of labour. The first stage of labour is primarily automatic; it is an involuntary body activity in the *growth, repair and reproduction* group of behaviours; behaviour that is linked to long-term survival. Too much stress will downgrade such activity and switch on short-term survival, *change the environment* behaviour.

A woman cannot will contractions. She has to accept them as they come and lose herself in them. In order for labour to progress smoothly, a mother must listen to the demands of her own body and act accordingly. If she feels pain, pain-avoidance behaviour should be switched on. Her mind must be in tune with her body.

This concept will be difficult to grasp for people who have not experienced childbirth. It is a totally new sensation to feel that one's body is taking such firm control of one's mind. Some women hate the feeling. It is annoying enough being unable to control the menstrual flow, but to be at the mercy of the far stronger uterine contractions in labour can be very disconcerting and unpleasant, particularly for humans who are used to exercising a far greater degree of mental control over their body than are animals.

Other women find contractions exciting and even enjoy them. Contractions can have a certain vitality which can be revelled in. They can give an experience of power and purpose which is wonderfully exhilarating. If each contraction can be welcomed instead of feared, then labour becomes an exciting job of work to do and there is an enormous feeling of satisfaction at a job well done. Labour can be immensely pleasurable in itself. The heightened awareness of the innate power of one's body can be a very enjoyable sensation and to deaden this feeling with pain relievers detracts greatly from the experience, which is described as sexually orgasmic by some women. After the long months of waiting for the baby to be born, it is wonderful to be able to participate fully in his birth.

In whatever way contractions are experienced, pleasant or unpleasant, at least something is happening. The knowledge that each contraction brings the birth itself that much closer is welcome indeed after nine long months of waiting.

Painfree contractions

It is very important to make a distinction between contractions and painful contractions. Contractions are not intrinsically painful, but can feel unpleasant or uncomfortable. The nearest comparison in most people's experience is the sensation that accompanies vomiting. Indeed, the process of vomiting also involves the contraction of smooth muscle and the expulsion of body cavity contents, this time of the digestive tract. Vomiting is uncomfortable and impossible to control, as are labour contractions, and one wishes that it were over, as many labouring women wish that their labour were over. But both stomach and uterine contractions must be endured rather than cured. The idea of taking a painkiller for vomiting is absurd. Moreover, if contractions are accompanied by pain, then cutting off pain perception in labour will also cut off the instinctive means of learning what to do to relieve the pain.

Painful contractions

There is no doubt that painful contractions of labour do occur. But pain is a motivation for the labouring woman to do something to ease her stress, whether physical or emotional. She may change her position to relieve physical stress and relax her body and mind to relieve psychological stress. Pain is motivation for pain-avoidance behaviour caused by specific biochemicals. After a few contractions, and in the absence of fear and panic, the labouring woman will learn that relaxation during contractions stops the pain. Pain increases stress hormone secretion which give an ACT *on your environment* command to the mind. In this instance the environment to be acted on is the position of the body itself and also the state of the mind.

Pain-avoidance behaviour is one of the basic instincts common to mammals. It is instinctive rather than innate, in that we have to learn how to avoid particular pains. For first-time mothers, contractions are a totally new experience but the onset of labour is gradual and by the time contractions become very strong, in a stress free environment, she will have learnt how to cope with them. Women should be given free rein to follow their instincts when dealing with contractions. If they are not allowed to follow their instincts, the pain will get worse because the underlying cause has not been dealt with.

Stress hormones tone down the strength of uterine contractions to give women time to learn how to cope with them. When the women has learnt that she must relax or change her position to avoid pain, then the uterus can get on with its work. The better she learns how to cope with contractions, to relax and follow positional instincts, the shorter will be the first stage of labour.

Freedom from pain depends on allowing uterine contractions to do their work without interference from the mind and the external environment. Painful contractions are an indication that labour is becoming less efficient. Pain slows labour by increasing ß-endorphin secretion. ß-endorphin is the biochemical cause of prolonged labour, also known as uterine inertia and dystocia. Prolonged labour is caused by physical and mental stress. If we can teach women how to reduce their stress levels then they can have painfree contractions. Enjoyable or uncomfortable? Yes or no, depending on mental attitude. Hard work? Certainly, no one has ever found a better word than labour. But intrinsically painful? No.

Relaxation for childbirth

Grantly Dick-Read's fear/tension/pain explanation of painful childbirth teaches that contractions are not necessarily painful but become painful if the woman becomes tense. Dick-Read was a fervent advocate of education for childbirth. He believed that once the link between fear and pain was understood then women could give birth naturally without fear and pain. He uncovered the physical effects of fear on the uterus but today his pioneering work is greatly undervalued. The fear of pain has not been eliminated, even with the wonders of modern anaesthetics. The fears of intervention and loss of dignity caused by cattle market obstetrics have been added.

The Lamaze system of childbirth is behavioural conditioning – psycho-prophylaxis. Women are taught to respond to contractions by relaxing skeletal muscle, to accept contractions instead of fighting them. This also is an effective way to deal with contractions. The net result of both Dick-Read's method and the Lamaze method is the same but psychoprophylaxis may have gained supremacy because it gives women something to do, a mental distraction, during contractions. On the other hand, the Lamaze technique is potentially stressful psychologically because it may itself be seen as a performance test and women may worry whether or not they are relaxing "properly".

First stage hormones

First Stage Oxytocin

Most women will know of oxytocin (Syntocinon) only as a drug used to augment labour when professionals consider that it is proceeding too slowly. Oxytocin is used to "cure" prolonged labour. But natural oxytocin is *not* secreted in large amounts during the first stage of normal labour.

Oxytocin can be thought of as petrol. While a car engine is running a small amount of petrol is used all the time – the engine can be revved while stationary. Similarly, oxytocin is secreted in small amounts all the time. But, however much petrol the engine receives, the car will not move with the handbrake on and the clutch depressed. In normal labour blood serum oxytocin remains at pre-labour levels throughout the first stage. Just as we do not to start to drive merely by putting our foot on the accelerator, labour does not start with increased oxytocin.

First stage contractions are initiated and spread at the level of the uterus itself rather than being directed from the brain. They are local contractions spreading locally through the action of prostaglandins. The low natural level of oxytocin is quite enough to lead to first stage contractions *if the uterus is ready to labour at all.* Contractions start not with higher blood levels of oxytocin, but with stretching of oestrogen-primed uterine muscle. The baby himself stretches the muscle. Stretching the cell changes its electrical activity making it more likely to respond to oxytocin.

Prostaglandins

The baby decides which cells to allow oxytocin to act on but, once a contraction has started, it spreads outwards by influencing adjacent cells with prostaglandin. Locally produced prostaglandin from contracting cells bypasses the need for blood oxytocin in adjacent cells.

The uterus is an engine with thousands of cylinders, and each cylinder is a muscle cell. Only when the action of all the cylinders is co-ordinated does the engine work at full power. However, unlike a petrol engine, where each cylinder must have its own supply of petrol, adjoining uterine muscle cells influence each other. Only a small group of cells need petrol to start a chain reaction of co-ordinated movement. If one contracts there will be a knock-on effect and adjacent cells may also contract.

Oxytocin is merely the first step in a biochemical chain reaction that leads to prostaglandin manufacture. Once one group of cells has made prostaglandins then the prostaglandin can diffuse locally and come into contact with adjacent cells. Whether or not the adjacent cells respond to this locally produced prostaglandin depends on whether they are oestrogen primed or ß-endorphin blocked – whether the hormonal clutch is depressed or raised.

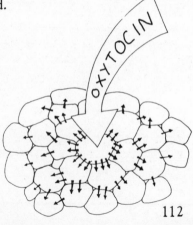

21: Oxytocin reaches a stretched uterine muscle cell and makes it produce prostaglandin which crosses to adjacent cells

Oxytocin and Oestrogen

Muscle cells need receptor sites for oxytocin in order to accept the *contract* message of oxytocin. Receptor sites for oxytocin are increased by exposing the uterus to oestrogen. Thus oestrogen sensitises the uterus to oxytocin. This is why oxytocin infusion alone is not always successful in inducing babies. If there are not enough receptor sites for oxytocin in the uterus then oxytocin alone will not turn a pregnant uterus to a labouring uterus. The *sensitivity* of the uterus to oxytocin is as important as the amount of circulating oxytocin in labour. Oestrogen increases oxytocin receptors. A labouring uterus is an oestrogen-primed uterus.

Met-enkephalin – another endorphin

The timing of contractions remains relatively constant. The initial oxytocin stimulus is released at three minute intervals from the mother's pituitary gland. This timing is achieved by a different endorphin regulator, met-enkephalin, which is a small section of the ß-endorphin molecule. Met-enkephalin is released from the same neurosecretory cells in the pituitary gland as oxytocin. Met-enkephalin lasts for about three minutes in the blood before being broken down and rendered ineffective.

Contractions start at three minute intervals towards the end of the first stage of labour. For those three minutes met-enkephalin has much work to do. It prevents further oxytocin release from the pituitary, it has pain-relieving powers and, like ß-endorphin, it prevents smooth muscle from contracting. Uterine muscle inhibition seems rather a paradox until one realises that, for co-ordinated labour contractions to be most effective, the full power of the uterus should be directed to the centre of the contraction initiated by the baby. Met-enkephalin may be found to quench the random uterine contractions that maintain muscle tone throughout pregnancy and between labour contractions. Scientists have already found evidence of the changing sensitivity of the uterus to met-enkephalin during pregnancy but are not yet aware of this possible function (Low et al, 1989). It is indeed possible that scientists have assumed erroneously that ß-endorphin cannot affect uterine contractions simply because they are aware of the co-secretion of oxytocin, a contraction promoting hormone, with a similar contraction stopping hormone, met-enkephalin.

Transition

Towards the end of the first stage, contractions become so powerful that each contraction seems to merge into the next with no respite in between. All this time the baby is gradually inching his way down towards the cervix. When he reaches the cervix and the gates are fully opened, he gives the order for the journey proper to begin.

Merely by passing through the cervix, the baby's head switches on hormonal instructions to release much greater supplies of oxytocin. The message is sent through nerves and so reaches the brain all but instantaneously. The baby's head has pressed the accelerator, but the mother is not yet aware of this great change.

The short time between the passage of the head through the cervix and the mother experiencing a strong urge to push is known as the transition stage. By stretching the cervix completely, the baby has already given the signal that the main part of the journey must start now. Stretching cervical and vaginal tissue sends a nervous signal (the neuropeptide hormone vasointestinal peptide, or VIP) directly to the mother's brain which switches on two hormonal instructions: release oxytocin and release prolactin. Some women are physically sick at this stage, our brains know before we do that we will shortly have to respond instinctively to push the baby out, and a flood of ACT hormone and ß-endorphin is also released. This stage is the transition between the passive acceptance of first stage contractions, for which we must be as relaxed as possible, and the active phase of labour when we have to use our voluntary abdominal and pelvic muscles to help our uterus expel the baby. It is an enormous behavioural transition.

Being a blood-carried message it takes time for the oxytocin to reach the uterus. But the behavioural effect of the oxytocin releasing hormone (VIP) on the brain is instantaneous. The feeling is very disorienting. A woman who has felt completely in control of her labour up to this point can suddenly becomes fey and appear to lose control completely. Her rational abilities seem to be non-existent. This stage feels a bit like the sensation of waking up knowing one is going to vomit and having just enough time to reach the bathroom before it is too late; only the feeling is far more intense and, for first-time mothers, there is no sense of foreknowledge of the next phase. Behaviour becomes totally instinctive: the woman may move like an automatum and change her position completely. At this point in my third labour I suddenly gave up and went to lie on the bed which was totally against my birth plan. I feel that this automatic position changing was directly caused by the position of my son's head as it passed through the cervix and that the birth position was chosen for me by my subconscious mind.

It is vitally important that the baby should enter the birth canal at the right angle. This is the most dangerous time of his journey and if he enters at an awkward angle the second stage may be slow. Maternal position is all important and should match as far as possible the foetal angle. The traditional practice of forcing women to deliver on their back so that attendants could see better what was happening must have caused countless deaths and vastly increased the need for forceps deliveries with the consequent risk of birth injury.

In a normal labour at this stage the next event is a flood of oxytocin reaching the uterus. The uterus reacts with a mighty shove, this time from the fundal muscle, which pushes the baby right through the cervix into the vagina. The vagina is supplied with sympathetic nerves. Now the mother knows her baby is very nearly born.

The Second Stage

The sensation of the baby in the birth canal demands instant action and ACT hormone is released along with ß-endorphin which masks much of what would be quite unbearable pain. ß-endorphin has a new role now – it must stop the uterus from careering out of control. ß-endorphin continues to tone down uterine contractions during the second stage of labour, this time by regulating oxytocin release – controlling the accelerator.

Timing is all important
- The baby's head passes through the cervix
- Stretch detectors in the cervix and vagina are activated
- A nervous signal (VIP) is sent to the pituitary gland to release oxytocin and met-enkephalin
- Oxytocin and met-enkephalin arrive at the uterus
- Fundal muscle pushes the baby through the cervix
- The baby's head impinges on vaginal sympathetic nerves
- The mother feels her baby for the first time as a truly independent being with a will of his own
- ACT hormone and ß-endorphin are secreted and the mother feels the urge to push

A few minutes later, perhaps even after the baby is born . . .
- A flood of ß-endorphin reaches the maternal circulation and acts on the uterus as a fail-safe device to prevent uterine rupture and to protect a foetus who is still in the birth canal from violent contractions.

The second stage is radically different from the first – both mentally and physically. Until now the uterus has been doing all the automatic subconscious work of drawing up the cervix and steering the foetus to the optimal position for the start of the journey down the vagina. The uterus now has a qualitatively different job to do: instead of merely changing its own shape to make an outlet for the baby, it has actively to propel and steer the baby downwards through the vagina. This is the most physically stressful part of labour for mother and baby alike, and both secrete large amounts of stress hormones to help them cope with it. The mother must co-ordinate her voluntary muscle activity with the involuntary uterine contractions to maximum effect and the baby, who is still relying on his mother's blood for oxygen, runs the risk of his blood supply being cut off during the journey because of compression of the cord against the cervix and vagina. It is amazing how well the baby can withstand this assault on his lifeline. He does not become brain-damaged until his supply of oxygen has been cut off for four minutes. A baby born with the cord tightly around him may be rather blue at birth but his stress hormones have directed available blood to where it is most needed – his brain. He has usually recovered from this assault by the time he is five minutes old. There is a popular belief that a baby can be strangled at birth by his own cord but it is compression of the cord that is dangerous rather than the cord being round his neck.

Unlike first stage contractions, which are initiated by the baby himself, second stage contractions probably do originate from the fundus, the largest and most powerful mass of uterine muscle (see figure 15, on page 92). The baby's head is now in the vagina and he is beyond the point where he can influence the uterus directly.

Ironically enough, although they are sceptical about the direction of the baby by the uterus in the first stage, which is fairly easy to understand in mechanical terms, obstetricians are agreed that the uterine forces direct and turn the baby as he passes through the vagina in the second stage where the direction must be achieved through nervous rather than purely mechanical means, a much more complicated method of control.

Having been physically (apart from at the uterus itself) and mentally relaxed for the first stage, the mother has to make a sudden switch from passively coping with contractions to the most physical active labour she and her uterus will do in her life. Suddenly the woman is aware for the first time that there is a real baby forcing its way out and that she must do all she can to help him on his way.

Second stage hormones
Oxytocin
Oxytocin is secreted as a response to stretch detectors in the cervix and in the vagina. As the baby passes these special cells he sends signals ordering more fuel for the journey. And as the baby presses against the nerves of the mother's sympathetic nervous system he tells the mother to push.

During the second stage, particularly at the placental site, oxytocin *reduces* the number of receptors for itself. It regulates its own action and is also regulated by ß-endorphin, both at the pituitary gland and at the uterus. High levels in the brain will prevent oxytocin secretion and high levels at the uterus reduce uterine muscle sensitivity to oxytocin.

For the second stage the mother's sympathetic pelvic nerves tell her that it is time to share control of birth with her uterus and she starts pushing in earnest. Oxytocin is telling her subconscious uterus to push and her voluntary sympathetic pelvic nerves are telling her voluntary muscles to push. She is suddenly aware of her child as a separate being who seems to be actively forcing his way out and requires her help. In reality the fundal muscle is pushing the baby downwards, but it feels as if the baby himself is pushing.

Throughout pregnancy and the first stage of labour the uterus has acted as a physical and psychological barrier between the woman and her child – the foetus might have been very active and kicked but these movements were muffled by the uterus, part of herself. But now the child himself impinges on her consciousness. He assumes a separate identity and is even more real to her than he was when first viewed on the ultrasound screen, and when he first kicked. The child has stopped being a parasite, taking what he needs passively through her body, and has started actively demanding attention. The second stage is the real start of motherhood. Hitherto, the mother has been a passive recipient of contractions but now she is called upon to ACT.

Bearing down
The urge to push is like the urge to defecate; nervous signals are virtually

indistinguishable between the two. This should come as no surprise to any woman who has acted on instinct in birthing her children. The only difference seems to be one of intensity. As I have mentioned before, we have had much practice in defecation and natural selection chose a similar process of evacuation for birth.

Unfortunately the urge to push is not always felt and acted on. The mother needs to co-ordinate her pushes with uterine contractions to ease her child gently into the world. But instinctive cues may so easily be masked. Some women may feel one long contraction and are unable to distinguish peaks, others may be too rigid in sticking to the taboo against defecating in public. Women undergoing epidural anaesthesia will not feel the bearing down instinct, and others may not be aware of it. Some women will be unable to find the right position, and some may be restrained on a delivery table, compelled to deliver against the forces of gravity. Old fashioned aids for the second stage were the birthing stool, a chair with a cut away seat, or a knotted sheet to pull on tied to the end of the bed. Modern aids include specially designed birthing chairs and delivery beds. Sometimes a full bladder causes delay but this can be emptied by catheterisation – even at home. If all else fails there are forceps and Ventouse vacuum extraction instruments.

The sensitive midwife comes into her own in the second stage. She can help the mother to co-ordinate her expulsive efforts with her uterine contractions. Rather than merely telling the mother what to do and when to push, she can breath with her and provide a constant stream of gentle reassurance that all is well. Empathy is more important than sympathy.

Birth

After a few pushes, the baby is born. This method of delivery is rather quaintly known as "maternal effort". Pushing the baby out does indeed hurt, but it is a soul cleansing hurt, a profound feeling of urgency, a deeply felt agony that seems to come from the depths of the soul or the very earth itself. It is one of the rare times in life when ecstasy and pain are almost indistinguishable. St Julian of Norwich described Christ's suffering on the cross in terms of the pangs of birth. New life comes through suffering and the new life makes the unbearable pain bearable. And then the mother can echo Christ's last words: "It is finished." The baby is born. A new life has come into the world.

The Third Stage

In the third stage of labour the placenta is expelled. This usually demands little effort on the mother's part and it is normal hospital practice to supply synthetic oxytocin coupled with a powerful contractant (Syntometrine) to enable the uterus to continue to contract until the uterus is empty. This medical management of the third stage of labour has caused problems in the past – there have been cases when an unexpected twin has been locked into the uterus, or part of the placenta has been retained. In nature oxytocin is supplied by the baby suckling. Suckling activates stretch receptors in the breasts which release oxytocin in exactly the same way as stretch detectors in the cervix and vagina. The baby roots for the breast as soon as he is born. Suckling is an innate reflex. He continues to activate stretch detectors for oxytocin release after his birth. Now that the cord is cut and the baby is no longer pumping ß-endorphin into the placenta, the placental site is freed from its hormonal block and can be expelled.

The baby's stress hormone levels are sky high, being born is a radical assault on the baby's stress hormone system which has been preparing for this very moment. The mother's stress hormones are also sky high; birth is extremely stressful physically and instinctive behaviour has overruled rational behaviour. But the need for fast action has passed, the mother has delivered her baby and is now free from the physical stress of contractions. At long last she can meet her baby face to face. There is a wonderful sense of achievement like nothing else she has ever experienced. She is on cloud nine. She is in a state of euphoria caused by natural opiates. Her baby shares her feelings. A new family is born.

This is the joy of natural childbirth.

6   Stress and Labour

Love's Labour's Lost

Shakespeare

I have a feeling that the last chapter must have sounded very alien to some mothers and to mechanically minded professionals. What about the pain of contractions and the endless asking "How much longer is there to go?" or "Am I allowed to push yet?". In instinctive, stress-free labour neither of these questions is necessary for the mother, and they are better not asked. If we wait patiently for the first stage to take its natural course, and if we move as our bodies tell us to, we will be given the answers unequivocally by our own brains when the time is right. The only person who knows when the time is right is the mother herself. Anything at all that stops a woman listening to the demands of her own body will slow down labour by cutting off instinctive cues and cutting down the supply of contraction-promoting hormones to the uterus. A sensitive midwife will help her to ease her baby gently into the world to minimise damage to the perineum but little other professional help should be required for birth itself. We already know how to deliver our babies ourselves. Nature has been selecting genes for natural childbirth since the year dot.

ß-endorphin in labour
Research studies show steadily rising levels of ß-endorphin throughout labour, both spontaneous and induced labour (Facchinetti *et al*, 1982). I suspect that the high levels found during labour have been one of the reasons why ß-endorphin is currently thought to have no effect on the uterus itself. The psychological function of ß-endorphin in labour is thought to be pain relief and its physical function has been completely overlooked.

If ß-endorphin is a contraction stopping hormone why are such high levels found in labour? High levels in pregnancy are predictable, prevention of co-ordinated contractions in pregnancy is all important, but what is the advantage of stopping contractions in labour itself?

ß-endorphin regulates labour
Labour is an explosive hormonal situation. Explosive situations are intrinsically dangerous. Contractions themselves spread by positive feedback signals – contractions release prostaglandin which in turn causes more contractions. More and more oestrogen is pumped into the uterus making it ever more sensitive to oxytocin. Positive feedback is responsible for explosive situations. Bombs are designed using positive feedback properties of explosives, and the uterus is designed to work using positive feedback properties of hormones.

Without the control of stress hormones, labour would inevitably lead to uterine rupture and foetal death. The uterus would contract so violently during

119

the second stage that the baby would be catapulted into the world like a bullet from a gun. The mother's cervix, perineum and vagina would be ripped to shreds.

The brain measures the physical and psychological stresses of the mother and rations labour hormones according to her ability to withstand physical stress, while taking into account her psychological needs. ß-endorphin regulates the supply of oestrogen in the first stage of labour and of oxytocin in the second. The more stress a mother experiences, the longer it will take to deliver the baby.

We have already come across higher stress hormone levels in pregnancy from various sources, the maternal hypothalamus and ovaries, the foetal pituitary, the placenta and the foetal membranes. Nearly all of these are effects of the regulation of reproduction by ß-endorphin, not psychological stress. How does one untangle these many reproductive sources of ß-endorphin and ACT hormone from another source – maternal psychological stress? We know that psychological stress and ß-endorphin have effects on ovulation. Is there any evidence supporting the ß-endorphin theory or is it fundamentally flawed simply because it is presented by a woman who happens to be a strong believer in home birth?

At present there is very little hard evidence that psychological stress impairs uterine function, or that raised ß-endorphin secretion is the cause.

The research literature on ß-endorphin and labour grows larger almost daily but no one seems to have given any attention at all to the psychological circumstances of ß-endorphin secretion. The key to uncovering the mysteries of labour has been available for seventeen years but no one has tried it in the lock before, although one of the pioneering researchers, Candace Pert, insisted on a home birth so that her baby could have his full share of ß-endorphin (Goldberg, 1990). ß-endorphin is the key. It opens two doors: the first the physical working of the uterus in labour and the second the psychology of labour. Physical and mental function are inextricably linked in childbirth.

Physical stress
We can expect to find raised ß-endorphin levels during labour itself because labour is an extreme physical stress and physical stress raises ß-endorphin secretion. Moreover, ß-endorphin regulates the secretion of oestrogen and oxytocin. If labour is to be efficient, smooth and safe for both mother and baby, we should expect to find finely tuned regulation of labour hormones. ß-endorphin regulates the potentially explosive situation of labour itself.

Since contractions are controlled automatically we are not allowed to take a break and have a rest as we would in other situations involving hard physical labour. ß-endorphin, secreted as a response to physiological stress, attempts to match the strength of contractions with our physical ability to cope with them. Without some automatic form of regulation the labouring uterus could go out of control and even rupture, with dire consequences for both mother and baby.

ß-endorphin acts to restrain the full power of the uterine engine all the way through labour. We cannot cut out ß-endorphin caused by physical stress except by using physical means to overcome physical barriers, for example allowing a woman to change her position at will, in response to her instinctive cues.

Labour is hard physical work. The only way to avoid this work completely is caesarean section, which brings long-term physical and psychological stress in its wake. We can, however, make each contraction a useful contraction. Much pain in labour is caused by forces of contractions being cancelled out by opposing forces from outside the body. If this happens there will be a see-saw effect between the opposing forces and instead of moving the baby downwards and thus changing the part of the uterus being stretched, the same part of the uterus may be constantly stretched, supplies of chemicals in the cells needed for contraction will be depleted, and pain will ensue.

Complete freedom of movement is essential in order to follow pain-avoidance instincts. Curtailing movement by connecting women up to drips and foetal monitors may be counterproductive and lead to the very pain and foetal distress it is meant to avoid. At least modern women are usually allowed to be mobile for the first stage of labour today. Forcing women to labour on their back must have been torture and in itself could account for a large proportion of infant and maternal mortality. Even today maternal exhaustion is often given as a reason for operative delivery – how much of that exhaustion has been caused by a poor understanding of the mechanism of labour? If we want to have shorter, less painful labours then we should do all we can to cut out physical stress.

Evidence

I have found no research papers on ß-endorphin secretion in natural labour so no one knows what constitutes normal levels. Many of the studies measuring ß-endorphin secretion in labour are fundamentally flawed because the mothers investigated were undergoing medical induction of labour and if labour is induced rather than spontaneous the theory predicts that ß-endorphin levels will be raised.

To give any true meaning to observed differences, stress hormone measurements have to be controlled for variations in daily rhythmical changes in stress hormone secretion. The easiest way to do this is to measure hormone levels in different patients at the same time of day. It is more convenient for researchers to study women whose labour is induced at 9 o'clock in the morning rather than to wait for women admitted in spontaneous labour in the middle of the night. Moreover, stress hormones levels may well be abnormally raised, with stress hormones induced by hospitalisation and medical intervention itself secreted on top of reproductive ß-endorphin. Almost by definition, intervention involves psychological stress because it takes control away from the patient. Patients awaiting surgery are known to suffer psychological stress and are given a pre-med, a tranquillizer, to calm them down before an operation. Women admitted for induction are likely to have higher stress hormone levels for psychological reasons because a woman whose labour is induced has already had a certain degree of control taken out of her hands and put into the hands of professionals. Quantitative assays are unable to measure *causes* of secretions. They will be unable to distinguish between ß-endorphin secreted as a response to the physical stress of labour itself, and that caused by psychological stress. A truer picture of ß-endorphin secretion could be found by measuring levels at term before labour is established and in spontaneous labour both at home and in hospital. This work has yet to be done because no one has realised its potential importance.

A few studies have measured ACT hormone secretion and, because ß-endorphin is secreted in parallel with ACT hormone, these studies give a hint of the effect of ß-endorphin.

Evidence from scientific experiments
If a labouring rat is handled after the birth of her first pup, the birth of the second pup is delayed. However, if she is handled but also given an anti-opiate drug, naloxone, the birth of the second pup is not delayed. This is a naloxone reversible effect of stress-induced ß-endorphin secretion and fully supports my predictions. (Leng *et al*, 1988).

Evidence from biochemistry
ß-endorphin works in the opposite way to both oestrogen and oxytocin. Oestrogen and ß-endorphin both have the same chemical hook to join on to oestrogen receptors on cells in the hypothalamus, and at the uterus as well (Low *et al*, 1989; Laniyonu, 1989). Oestrogen links uterine cells together electrically. ß-endorphin raises the electrical potential of cell membranes making them less likely to respond to contraction promoting hormones. Oxytocin reduces cell membrane potentials. Smooth muscle cells need calcium to contract. ß-endorphin reduces the amount of free calcium in a cell. Oxytocin frees calcium.

Evidence from drugs
It is accepted that adrenaline slows labour and there is also evidence that opiate drugs interfere with uterine function. General side effects of opiates are listed in the *British National Formulary* (March 1989): "Opioid analgesics share many side-effects though qualitative and quantitative differences exist. *They all cause constipation (by reduction of intestinal motility), respiratory depression, cough suppression, urinary retention, nausea,* and tolerance [my italics]." Most of these effects are depressive effects on smooth muscle. Why should the uterus be the only organ where the effect is not seen? It is not. Pethidine, a synthetic opiate slows down labour.

When I was discussing my ß-endorphin and stress theory with an obstetrician he thought that there might be something in the theory because giving diamorphine to women whose labour stopped on arrival in hospital sometimes restarted contractions. This seemed a body blow for the theory; opiates should not restart contractions but further prolong labour. However, in the *British National Formulary* we find the following entry: "Diamorphine (heroin) is a powerful opioid analgesic. It is more likely to produce euphoria and addiction than morphine but causes relatively *less nausea, constipation,* and hypotension [my italics]." In other words the relaxing effects on the mind are stronger than the depression of smooth muscle activity. Relaxing the mind with diamorphine reduces stress-induced ß-endorphin secretion enough to allow labour to restart. But how much better to avoid the stress in the first place.

Evidence from clinical observations

Anecdotal evidence about psychological stress in labour abounds but scientists want hard facts. There is a very large gap in the research literature about psychological stress in labour - just nine papers out of 1,500,000 or more medical research papers published in the last five years dealt specifically with psychological stress and labour and two of those papers dealt with the stress of birth attendants rather than stress of the mother herself (*Index Medicus* 1988-June 1992). Medical scientists are just not interested in stress in normal labour, indeed, I would go so far as to say that they are not interested in normal labour at all.

Paradoxically, some of the best evidence for the role of stress in labour comes from a Dublin hospital renowned for active management of labour with 40% of labours accelerated by oxytocin infusion. This hospital manages to combine a high rate of intervention with a low rate of caesarean section - less than 4% (O'Driscoll and Meagher, 1986). This seems to be a body blow for the view that medical intervention causes stress interfering with normal labour. In Dublin active management is given the credit for low caesarean rates but other factors may be much more important. Antenatal education is excellent, and antenatal education itself is a tacit acknowledgement that the mother's mind has a role to play in labour. Mothers are constantly attended by midwives, not monitored by faceless machines. Mothers are kept fully informed as to their treatment. Because nursing sisters are given more authority than junior doctors, and also active management of labour adheres to a strict set of rules, there are less likely to be whispered arguments between staff at the mother's bedside. All these conditions prevent panic, panic of staff and of patients and panic is a classic cause of an increased stress hormone response. Indeed O'Driscoll himself recognises this.

Obstetricians implementing active management of labour in Great Britain have been unable to duplicate Dublin's low caesarean section rates, most probably because they think of active management only in terms of drug treatment and leave out psychological measures such as the continuous attention of a midwife.

Dr Vernon Coleman cites a research paper in the *New England Journal of Medicine* which showed that providing women with a constant unqualified companion for the duration of labour reduced the average length of labour from around nineteen hours to just eight hours. Psychological support is so important for labouring women that it can eliminate prolonged labour at a stroke.

Psychological Stress

As recently as 1991 Derek Llewellyn Jones stated in his basic textbook for medical students:

"It must be confessed that although it is agreed that emotions may affect uterine activity, the mechanism of their effect is not known."

The mechanism of the effect on labour by the emotions is exactly the same as the physiological mechanisms controlling labour itself. High ß-endorphin regulates labour and even higher ß-endorphin caused by psychological stress prolongs it to the point where it becomes dangerous.

Pregnant women have been attending relaxation classes for decades yet the professionals still appear not to know why relaxation helps in childbirth, and many obstetricians continue to be sceptical. Psychological stress is subjective and therefore notoriously difficult to measure scientifically and yet most people have an idea of what is meant by psychological stress, even pure scientists. Scientists know how to inflict such stress on animals and the stresses are largely similar in humans. Animal lovers seem to know more about the stresses of laboratory animals than many maternity professionals know about the psychological stresses of labouring women. Relaxation can be defined as an absence of stress, both physiological and psychological, and therefore an absence of stress-induced ß-endorphin.

To return to the analogy with driving a car, the mother controls the progress of labour according to the environmental hazards she encounters. The more hazards she has to deal with, the slower the journey. It is not always safe to drive too slowly, it can make other drivers take unnecessary risks. Slow labour can indeed exhaust the mother and overstress the foetus and lead to foetal and maternal death. What then is the selective advantage of allowing psychological stress to interfere with labour?

Let me recap on the behavioural purposes of stress hormones. They are switched on in an attempt to make us change the environment to suit our needs better. Once our needs are met then stress hormones fall, and the body resumes its normal activity. The evolutionary purpose of psychologically induced stress hormones in labour is to improve the environment to make it more suitable for labour, for birth itself, and for welcoming a new person into the world.

The right environment for labour

Fear

We are more prone to psychological stress than animals because we have culture, foresight, imagination and education. Man's accumulated experience is part of his mental environment. The accumulated experience of childbirth since man became civilised and started to share more knowledge has been predominantly characterised by pain and disaster. Gordon Bourne is indeed right to castigate women for spreading horror stories about childbirth, but the medical profession must share the blame. Simply redefining childbirth as a medical emergency that needs hospital treatment increases the fear that is already part of our culture. The fear of childbirth itself leads to inefficient uterine function leading to pain and more fear, leading to more stress. A vicious circle.

Hospital or home?

The environment is of paramount importance to the labouring woman. In a stressful environment stress hormones inhibit the normal working of the uterus. As a general rule, new situations are stressful situations. The more familiar a woman is with a place, the less stress she will feel in it. Familiar people and routines will cause less stress than strange people and strange routines. One major problem in hospitals is that professionals, who are familiar with the place and procedures will underestimate the stress induced by the hospital itself as well as the psychological stresses of medical treatment. Professionals may not realise just how alien hospitals are to most people; indeed many people have an instinctive fear of hospitals, associating them with pain and death. Professionals are familiar with hospital routine treatments, nurses may set up intravenous drips every day of their working lives, but for the patient this may be a novelty and therefore intrinsically frightening.

A woman's environment includes not only bricks and mortar but the presence of other people and her relationship with them. The more sympathetic they are towards her the better she will be able to cope, the more domineering and powerful they are, the more her stress hormones will rise. Even sympathy is not enough, empathy, which is feeling with her rather than for her, is best.

Sensitive midwives advise women not to go into hospital too early. They know all too well that labour is likely to slow down once the mother arrives in hospital. The onset of labour and a normal first stage both depend on low stress hormone levels. The first stage of labour will proceed most efficiently when maternal ß-endorphin levels are low. Relaxation, freedom of movement and freedom from psychological stress are all important for the first stage of labour.

The biological function of stress hormones in the first stage of labour is to enable a woman to reach a safe place for delivery and birth. Slowing down labour gives the woman time to return to the nest. Unfortunately, most women use this time to travel to hospital which, despite the best efforts of the establishment, is not the safest place for birth except for a very small number of women (those with a phenotypically, as opposed to genetically, small pelvis and women with a low placenta, both of which will require a caesarean section). However, there is no doubt that hospital is perceived as the safest place for birth by most women and at least the detrimental effects of fear are partly overcome. Improved pain relief has also reduced the fear of pain. These two factors removing fear may themselves account for improved mortality rates in the past decade.

Improving the environment

Hospital childbirth is becoming a little more consumer oriented, but hospitals are still a million miles away from providing the labouring woman with what she needs most - freedom from stress and freedom to control her own labour. Hospital environments have become marginally less threatening but much more could be done to make hospital birth less stressful. It is no good professionals trying to decide what improvements to make. Hospital is their work place, their second home and their experience of the hospital environment is radically different. Groups such as AIMS and ARM (the Association for Improvements in the Maternity Services, and the Association of Radical Midwives) have already done much research and have already outlined what improvements women want, but no one seems to listen. Women want more choice, more continuity in care - for example, seeing the same midwife for antenatal care and labour. They want more control over their own labours. All these improvements would lower ß-endorphin secretion in labour. Women might not know the science behind stress and labour; they may not know that stress itself interferes with normal labour; but they do know by intuition how labour could be improved.

Conclusions

In summary, psychological stress impedes labour at all stages. Stress leads to weak, unproductive contractions which may well exhaust both mother and baby. Unfortunately it will take decades before the obstetricians catch up with the pure research or admit to themselves that hormones can affect humans just as much, if not more, than they do animals. The basic scientific elements of this admittedly radical theory are founded in the last fifteen years of pure biochemical and endocrinological research. The psychological elements have been found mainly from personal experience, from anecdotal material in the midwifery and lay childbirth literature, and also fictional accounts of birth by contemporary authors such as Margaret Drabble in *The Millstone* and Lynn Reid Banks in *The L-Shaped Room*. Dick Francis is very perceptive about the physical effects of stress hormones in men - perhaps because he was a jockey and therefore more aware of his body and its reactions to stress.

The theory fits the facts as they are known at present and should lead to a radically different approach to childbirth. This hypothesis about the physical role of ß-endorphin in labour gives scientific foundation to female intuition during labour and it teaches us the paramount importance of following our instincts - including our instincts regarding place of labour.

ß-endorphin block hypothesis

I have called this theory the "ß-endorphin block hypothesis" and it follows directly onwards from the progesterone block hypothesis of Csapo which was presented in the 1960s. There are very many ways in which the hypothesis can be tested but most of this work is yet to be done. Until it is done I have no doubt that many people, particularly professionals, will remain sceptical but I feel that there is already enough solid scientific research material to justify using this theory as a working hypothesis in the management of normal labour. In any event, it is important that women themselves should know how stress slows labour in order for them to decide for themselves how to prevent stress during labour and how to deal with it should it arise.

Much more research needs to be done into practical ways of reducing stress. Traditional medicine is still very much biased towards repairing damage done by stress rather than searching out the root causes of stress. Stress reduction research does not attract funds from drug companies because it would reduce consumption of drugs like tranquillizers and sleeping pills. There are no fortunes to be made in preventing ill health – only profits to be lost.

Complementary medicine has gone a lot further along the road than conventional medicine, which remains rooted in a reductionist view of the human body, seeing organs and processes in isolation from the rest of the body, a view which is reflected by the increasing specialisation of medical disciplines. Complementary medicine already understands the importance of links between the mind and the body.

Relaxation, breathing methods, yoga and psychoprophylaxis have all proved successful means of dealing with stress in labour by screening out distractions, and many mothers and midwives will testify to their efficacy. Until now, the reasons for the success of these methods have been unknown. Home birth remains the only way for a woman to be sure of retaining control over her baby's birth and I recommend it highly as an experience not to be missed unless absolutely necessary.

THE
HUMANITY
OF
CHILDBIRTH

7   *Childbirth in History*

"The care of women during childbirth has been described as a measure of the degree of civilisation of a community."

W.T.W Nixon, former Professor of Obstetrics and Gynaecology in *Childbirth*, Penguin

The Dangers of Civilised Childbirth

Civilisation itself is the principal cause of 99% of the problems encountered in childbirth barring those purely of genetic origin. The human body has not yet adapted to the civilised existence; natural selection cannot work fast enough to cope with the swift environmental changes wrought by culture. The advent of cooking changed man's diet at a stroke – he ate less raw fruit and foliage, and more meat thus failing to obtain enough essential vitamins. There is considerable evidence that spina bifida is caused by folic acid deficiency in the first six weeks of pregnancy while the foetus' spine is being formed (folic acid is found in leafy foods). I have no doubt that other birth defects will be found to be owed to dietary deficiencies. Women inherit genetic instructions for safe childbirth but nutritional factors can lead to poorly developed physique and a deformed pelvis. More importantly, society's complete ignorance of the fact that childbirth is a natural instinctive event rather than a medical emergency leads to psychological failings.

The causes of problems in childbirth are many and varied: universal fear of childbirth spread by the spoken and written word; poor living conditions; malnutrition leading to poor development; inadequate sanitation and water supplies leading to disease; and the suppression of natural instincts during labour. The Welfare state and modern hospital-based obstetrics have relieved some problems but compounded others; however, it would be grossly unfair to lay all the blame at the door of the obstetrician. As mankind has become ever more civilised, women and children have suffered. Western society itself is suffering the consequences of trying to take over control of reproduction from nature, with dire effects on the quality of family life and society as a whole.

Physical factors

Civilisation itself has reduced our efficiency in childbearing. We moved away from the countryside and congregated in large settlements where there was a lack of fresh water and fresh food. Waste disposal was a major problem. Insanitary arrangements attracted rats which spread disease. We no longer lived off the land but had to rely on food brought in from outside the city which meant inevitable shortages from time to time and resulted in an unbalanced diet, particularly for the poor. With slow transport and no refrigeration often the food had started to rot before it was eaten; or it was

131

preserved with salt or, more recently, sugar, reducing its food value and leading to more imbalance. We began sitting on chairs instead of squatting on our heels and thus reduced the flexibility of the pelvis. We invented beds and took to them in childbirth, so turning a natural function into an illness. We became embarrassed and inhibited about natural bodily functions. We fed our babies on cow's milk instead of breastmilk, nature's contraceptive, and wore ourselves out with childbearing.

As we moved away from the countryside we had fewer chances to marvel at the natural childbirth of domestic animals. We lost faith in our ability to give birth and learnt to ignore our instincts. History was written by city-dwellers who saw only civilised birth which was dangerous and painful. They concluded that birth was always thus, and so the myth of a woman's sorrow in childbed was born, teaching us all to fear childbirth. The fear made us tense, and the tension led to pain and yet more pain as stress hormones interfered with the body's natural functioning. We were content with midwives and their natural remedies for five millennia but eventually the doctors arrived on the scene, saving a few lives with their new-fangled forceps but also bringing with them more pain and death.

Meanwhile, back at the farm, children grew up in large extended families – many hands were needed to till the soil before the advent of the agricultural revolution. Birth and death were everyday occurrences; children would grow up seeing domestic animals being born and would care for orphan lambs in the spring as well as helping their mother care for their young siblings. Such familiarity with birth and death would leave less room for fear, which usually results from ignorance. There were no books to repeat tales of disaster and to lead to an expectation of pain. The oft-repeated tale of a woman in a far away place taking an hour or two away from work to deliver her child and then returning to continue her work with the new baby swaddled close to her would have been typical in an agricultural society. Childbirth was all in the day's work. Life was hard, women could not afford the luxury of taking time off work and treating childbirth as an illness. The labour of childbirth was not so very much harder than the labours of everyday life. Although pregnant women were slowed down by their placidity and extra bulk there was still work to be done and a family to feed. Later on, labour was welcomed as heralding a respite from everyday domestic chores; family and neighbours would rally round to care for the rest of the family during the lying-in time.

There were no professionals to call upon and indeed little need for them; the collective experience of women and men in the small community, gleaned over the years from human and animal labours, sufficed to see a woman through labour. She already had much experience in childcare, and breastfeeding came naturally, aided by experience of milking domestic animals. Natural selection continued to weed out mistakes but death was closer to life in those days and therefore feared less. This was no peaceful rural idyll but the hard life of the frontier between savagery and civilisation, an era when man had done little to ease the relentless struggle for life.

Later on the gentleman farmer's wife had a bad time during labour. She was utterly unaccustomed to hard domestic labour, being allowed the indulgence of servants to do the heavy work thereby rendering her body less fit for the hard physical labour of childbirth that was to come. She was better educated, could read the Bible, and learned that she would bring forth her children in sorrow. The original mistranslation of the seventeenth century is still being perpetuated even by obstetricians sympathetic to the need to keep labouring women free from stress (Burns, 1992).

Childbirth became an illness. The gentlewoman took to her bed for labour and discovered pain. Her husband, in his anxiety for his delicate wife, called for the doctor, his drugs and his instruments rather than for the midwife, who was in a lower social class and therefore unfit to attend to his wife. Neither she, her husband nor the doctor ever asked that most important question – why did she feel pain when her poorer sisters did not? If the question was ever asked the answer was assumed to be "superior breeding" – quite the opposite answer to that predicted by evolutionary theory!

Most contemporaneous accounts of childbirth were written by educated women who had a terrible time in childbirth. They were brought up to think they were dainty creatures, too refined to acknowledge their animal origins. It was unseemly for a married lady even to enjoy sex; intercourse was an unpleasant requirement of marriage to be passively endured. Childbirth must have come as an appalling physical and mental shock to these women; they had to learn to lie down and think of England during childbirth as well as during sex. It is no wonder that they fought for the right to pain relief and handed their children over to nursemaids at the earliest opportunity.

Childbed

Childbirth was called childbed until the last century; women were expected to take to their beds during labour, and this served only to complicate matters further and to increase the pain. Confinement in bed grossly disrupts the interactive dance between the uterus and foetus. A woman whose movement is greatly restricted will be unable to change her position at will to avoid pain and thus to move as her instincts dictate – if she allows herself to be instinctive at all. Social training for gentlewomen militated against anything so distasteful.

The baby cannot be guided into the best position for his final journey with his mother flat on her back. He passes through the cervix at the wrong angle which leads to problems in the second stage of labour. These problems had utterly appalling consequences; before the invention of forceps babies could be stuck in the vagina for hours at a time. This cut off blood supply to the back passage and destroyed tissue between the vagina and rectum. After such a birth a woman had to live with perpetual uncontrollable leakage of faeces from her vagina and often became a social pariah (Dally, 1991). During the second stage of labour the supine mother is actually pushing her baby out against the forces of gravity. The human pelvis is an adaptation from the quadruped pelvis for bipedalism, nature carefully tucked the coccyx out of the way as far as possible only for civilisation to allow it to interfere again. Many women died in childbed or survived with terrible injuries.

The Industrial Revolution

The coming of the industrial revolution brought more people to the cities to face poverty, malnutrition, overwork and disease. Childbirth became even more dangerous and yet women still lived to produce large numbers of children, even if half of them were stillborn or died in infancy. For women having to combine work outside the home with pregnancy and childcare, a life of overwork, malnutrition and starvation wages conspired to ensure that the milk soon dried up along with its contraceptive properties. Even the railways played their part in worsening the situation by bringing in supplies of unpasteurised milk from the surrounding countryside for city babies. This led to earlier weaning, the withdrawal of the immunological protection of mother's milk and the risks of contaminated feeding equipment leading to higher infant mortality. A breastfeeding mother will not usually ovulate until the baby is at least six months old, so earlier weaning meant more babies. (The period of natural contraception varies from society to society depending on factors such as maternal nutrition and the age of the child when weaned.)

The horrors of childbirth and motherhood in the last century and early in the twentieth century are well documented in an eye-opening book, *Maternity*, a collection of 160 accounts of motherhood written by working women and first published in 1915. The link between nutrition, overwork, large families and poverty is proved very clearly and I recommend the book to anyone sceptical about the causes of death before hospitalised childbirth. Mothers were the first ones to suffer when families were poor and, out of an income averaging less than 25s a week (£1.25) they scrimped, saved and starved themselves to find the doctor's fee of five guineas (£5.25) for the birth itself. The accounts written by women who were financially better placed are in stark contrast to their poverty stricken sisters – they write mostly about their ignorance of the facts of life, contraception and labour and the problems thus caused.

Mothers and children were forced to work long hours in factories to scrape together enough money to live and this only added to the toll of sickness. Such a hard life meant that people simply could not afford the time to help neighbours out in times of need; professionals were called in for childbirth. Middle class ladies with too much time on their hands went about doing good and the seeds of today's charities were planted.

Hospitals

It has been said that the Victorians solved problems by throwing bricks at them. They built workhouses for the poor, hospitals for the sick and asylums for the mentally ill. The sewer building and water works probably did far more than anything else to alleviate human illness; taking people away from their homes in times of sickness was often counterproductive. Anaesthesia had been invented and surgery was all the rage. The status of doctors and surgeons increased as the middle classes expanded. Childbirth was a lucrative source of income in the days of large families. But the budding surgeon obstetricians needed a constant supply of labouring women on which to practice in order to exploit this new vein of gold. The Victorians started to build lying-in hospitals.

Childbirth was now so dangerous that it was impossible to see it as a natural process. The first women to use the new hospitals were not the rich middle classes but the charity cases, unmarried mothers and those too poor even to afford the services of the local midwife. These mothers went through agony, strapped down lying on their backs with their legs in the air – a real punishment for the sins of poverty and fornication. Many died of childbed fever introduced by the infected hands of the doctors themselves. The maternal and perinatal death rates soared for women delivered in hospital, so much so that Florence Nightingale wrote that: "Not a single lying-in woman should ever pass the doors of a general hospital" (Pearsall, 1971). A century later, with the advent of aseptic techniques, safer caesarean section and antibiotics, death rates have plummeted but are Florence Nightingale's words still pertinent today?

I believe that they are. Hospital childbirth is dangerous even before any intervention takes place because it saps self-confidence and undermines natural instincts. Unfortunately most Western women are now in the unenviable position of the gentleman farmer's wife who took to her bed for childbirth and let the doctor take over. The dangers of childbirth are drummed into us by the medical establishment, hospital treatment is supposed to save us from danger, pain and suffering; but we continue to hear dreadful stories. Women still tend to compare horror stories of hospital birth instead of recounting the joys. Why is birth still such a disaster area? Why are advocates of natural childbirth dismissed as masochistic earth mothers? And what is natural childbirth?

Instinctive Childbirth

Since childbirth is a natural bodily function, finely tuned by natural selection before man acquired consciousness, women should give full rein to their instincts rather than attempting to let the mind rule the body. Consciousness, culture, foresight and social pressures have disrupted physical and hormonal instinctive cues in labour to such a degree that civilised childbirth has automatically become painful and dangerous. Nature took pains to free the pregnant and labouring woman from the interference of her socially conditioned behaviour. ß-endorphin and ACT hormone levels are raised in pregnancy and labour and the evolutionary significance was to ensure that woman's blossoming verbal and symbolic reasoning abilities did not make her forget her biological purpose – which was the perpetuation of her genes.

Intuition – the sixth sense
Natural selection allowed the male to lose more of his sixth sense, intuition, because he played a smaller role in childcare. If anything, a finely developed sixth sense denotes intellectual superiority, but intuition is seen as irrational in a patriarchal society because it is something that most men lack rather than because it denotes intellectual inferiority. The sixth sense is a qualitatively

different type of reasoning. Verbal reasoning is thinking with words, and non-verbal reasoning is thinking in symbols. Science is limited to answering questions phrased in words or symbols and thus concentrates almost exclusively on verbal and symbolic reasoning. Merely trying to express in words thoughts arrived at through intuitive reasoning presents a problem in itself – a problem which has dogged me throughout the writing of this book.

Significant breakthroughs in scientific thought have been made by scientists freeing themselves from the constraints of so-called logical reasoning. Intuitive reasoning is not constrained by having to define problems in terms of words or symbols before working out how to solve them. Intuitive reasoning is akin to Edward de Bono's lateral thinking, and can solve problems directly without having to translate them first into words. I think that intuitive reasoning is elicited by stress hormones. The more stressed we are, the more our brain tries to solve problems causing stress. Flashes of inspiration are sixth sense intuitions and often occur when people are under stress caused by overwork, tiredness and danger. They can induce scientists to ask new questions and solve previously insoluble problems. People sleep on problems to let their subconscious brain solve problems that are not amenable to verbal and symbolic reasoning. We even call this sixth sense intuition "sensitivity" and it is seen as a primarily female trait. Sensitive men are often not "macho" enough to succeed in a patriarchal society. Sensitivity is seen as belonging to the arts rather than the sciences and this is why I think it has been a terrible mistake to label childbirth as a science instead of an art and to put labouring women in hospital.

In the environment of the hospital, instinctive behaviour is seen as emotional and is therefore labelled as irrational and inappropriate. The scientific doctor sees instinctive behaviour as irrational and intrinsically bad; he is frightened of it simply because it is not amenable to verbal and symbolic reasoning and he cannot fit it into his scientific frame of reference. Female professionals trained in the patriarchal model of scientific childbirth have been taught to disparage it, whereas radical midwives are far more aware of the importance of instinct in childbirth. The role of stress hormones in labour shows that it is vitally important that women should follow their instincts to reduce stress hormone levels. Instinctive behaviour during pregnancy and labour, so often derided in books on childbirth, was itself a positive selection force in evolution. Nature designed the childbirth mechanism long before she gave us verbal and symbolic reasoning abilities and she seems to have taken some trouble to screen out these ill-effects of consciousness. Most medical textbooks and handbooks intended for the general public are full of references to women's putative irrationality during pregnancy. Gordon Bourne writes:

"Even the most highly competent and efficient woman may find that her judgement is impaired. She may be inclined to make hasty decisions, her reasoning may not be as rational as it would normally be and her conclusions may be inaccurate and incorrect...

"There is no doubt that the nervous system is more sensitive during pregnancy

making women seem almost unreasonable and occasionally they will not even respond to logical argument."

This irrationality is generally seen by doctors as something to be guarded against for the woman's own good or, if that argument fails to impress her, for the sake of her baby. However, there is no need for a woman to use powers of intellectual reasoning during labour, her body should tell her what to do and when – the irrationality of pregnancy is a preparation for the birth itself.

Women do not *lose* their ability to reason at all but have stronger intuitions – a better sixth sense. This insight, being subconscious and controlled by prelinguistic centres of the brain, is difficult to put into words which perhaps accounts for it being labelled irrational. But it is *pre-rational* rather than irrational.

We have not lost the instincts pertaining to childbirth, but hospital childbirth teaches us to ignore or mistrust them; instinct is ignored and belittled in the hospital setting. There are countless tales of women in despair in hospitals, forced to submit to routine practices totally at odds with their instinctive wishes. One obstetrician gives positive instructions to his staff never to let a mother close her eyes during labour. She is not even allowed to escape into her own mind during labour but must let the doctors do her thinking for her (O'Driscoll and Meagher, 1986).

Conclusion

Hospital childbirth brought yet more pain, death and suffering, caused directly by intervention in an instinctive event. Although professionals claim to have dealt with the pain and the death, the suffering continues. Human childbirth has been intrinsically dangerous and painful since the dawn of civilisation because of the advent of fear and the denial of instincts. In past eras a civilised lifestyle was an unhealthy lifestyle owing to overcrowding, poor sanitation, disease, malnutrition and poverty, all of which produced unhealthy women with malformed bodies. It is a wonder that the human race survived at all. Today most of the problems of poor physique have been eliminated, but the dangers of fear and a passive approach to childbirth remain.

8   Medicalised Childbirth

"Conventional Childbirth

"In this choice, the woman is admitted to the maternity ward in the currently conventional way... She is content to leave the process of childbirth in the care of the obstetric team, and to accept, without question, their management. She may or may not be told why a procedure takes place, and usually does not want her partner to support her during childbirth. She is cared for with skill but does not participate in the process of childbirth."

Llewellyn-Jones, 1990

Social Pressure

Man is a social animal. Nature has designed us to be at ease with ourselves only when we conform to the behaviour expected by the social group. The biological temptation to act like sheep is enormous. When it comes to choosing where to have our babies we behave like lemmings and rush into hospital with all its inherent dangers. Women choosing to labour at home are seen by their peers as very brave but slightly addled in the brain. It takes a lot to resist peer pressure.

It takes even more to resist pressure from authority figures. We are brought up to respect doctors, to regard them as pure altruists who, like our parents, have only our best interests at heart. We respect their superior education, their vastly increased experience of medical conditions. It is difficult to say no to anything they prescribe. Obstetricians have a further weapon up their sleeves. If they fail to convince us of the need for treatment, they can play on our fears and insist on the treatment for the sake of our unborn child. The few women who manage to have a home birth today are regarded with deep suspicion by staff, who despise them, thinking that they put personal satisfaction before the health of their baby.

Birth plans
Despite the quotation at the beginning of this chapter, the birth plan is now given official status in some hospitals, although whether or not it is respected is another matter entirely. Birth plans include such options as type of pain relief required, position for the first stage of labour, whether the baby's father is to be present, whether the baby is to be bathed before being given to his mother, whether or not the mother wishes to breastfeed and so on. But all too often women arriving at hospital with detailed birth plans are regarded as a nuisance because hospital routines are not geared to giving women real choices. Birth plans can be overruled at any stage "for the sake of the baby".

Hospitals do not really want women to control their own labours, the official birth plan is little more than a sop to consumer demands for more choice in childbirth. But women need to be able to control their own labours because stress hormones that prolong labour are secreted in circumstances of lack of control. Dr Vernon Coleman writes that aggressive patients, those least liked by hospital staff, recover more quickly from surgery, and I suspect, from birth too. Aggressive patients are often those who want to retain control over their own bodies and health care whereas passive patients all too easily slip into a state of dependence – learned helplessness.

Self-confidence
Hospital childbirth saps self-confidence from the word go by teaching us that we cannot labour properly by ourselves. The more interventions that take place, the more helpless we feel, the more our self-confidence is drained and the less control we have over our own bodies. Stress hormones are increased in circumstances of helplessness, hopelessness and lack of control. A woman controlling her own labour must therefore control her physical and psychological environment.

Psychological stress and hospital childbirth
Hospitals are stressful by definition. Nothing can make them feel as safe as home. I could not help but laugh at a study comparing "simulated" home confinement in hospital with standard hospital controlled labour (there was little difference in outcomes). A home is a place where the host makes the rules and strangers have to toe the line or are made to feel unwelcome. Wallpaper, curtains, divans and soft music do not constitute even a simulated home. It takes time to settle into a new place and that time will prolong labour. Unless staff are familiar and trusted they cannot even start to become friends; moreover, building a friendship is time consuming and takes two. Staff on a busy labour ward lack both time and inclination for friendship. Even in a "simulated" home staff must maintain a professional distance from their patients; they are answerable not to their patients but to their professional superiors. To be accepted into their environment we must learn their code of behaviour and then follow it.

In recent years there have been very real attempts to break down barriers and turn the patient back into a human being but old habits die hard and the fact remains that patients will always be seen as intruders in the hospital environment and staff must continue to keep them at arm's length. The amount of mental energy needed to build a real relationship with each patient would be emotionally exhausting and vastly increase the nervous breakdown rate of hospital staff. Psychiatrists have the highest suicide rates amongst doctors for this very reason. Staff have to develop coping strategies when dealing with illness throughout their working lives, but few pregnant women are ill and hospital treatment is therefore inappropriate. Women giving birth in hospital must fight to maintain control of their own labour when all their mental energy is needed for labour itself. Babies are better born at home where there is no set system to battle against and the midwife attends by invitation, as a welcome guest and friend.

The hospital environment

Hospital is just about the worst place in which to give birth. Not only is hospital not home and therefore intrinsically stressful, but hospital is a second home for all those who work there, the patient is a guest and must follow the house rules of her host. The hospital is a normal environment for doctors, nurses, midwives and ancillary staff but a grossly abnormal environment for ordinary people. The staff are like a large self-contained family; they already know their own positions in the hierarchy, the geography of the site, the routines, the unwritten rules. The patient is an intruder who must be kept in her place.

Whenever I have been in hospital the only people with whom I could relate were other patients and the cleaners who, being at the bottom end of the pecking order themselves, were closest to my lowly position in the hierarchy. Even the language is different: birth is parturition, lying-in is the puerperium, stitches are sutures, urination is micturition. Medical language maintains a professional distance between the patient and those caring for her – it is a way of not allowing patients to infiltrate the hospital family. Medical language keeps the ignorant uninformed and humiliates those better informed by providing language traps to fall into. Nurses are go-betweens who act as translators for the doctors and thus preserve the doctor's position in the hierarchy. Doctors resent too much knowledge in a patient because it detracts from their professional self-esteem. But pregnant women are notorious for wanting to know all about labour. This is one reason why they are particularly prone to argue with their obstetrician, and run the risk of becoming labelled as problem patients. Another reason is the secretion of testosterone towards the end of pregnancy which makes women more aggressive and ready to fight to protect their young, as yet unborn.

While we are encouraged to read certain rather patronising books on pregnancy and labour, we are warned against reading too much for our own good. It is never a good idea to wave books at doctors in an attempt to make them change their proposed treatment for any problem; their views will become more entrenched and the possibility of a change of heart will recede further into the distance. Management of labour then becomes a battle of wills, and because staff are in the strongest position, they usually win. Fortunately, consent forms are a necessary part of hospital life and the patient always retains the right to say "no".

Pressures to conform

We have an innate and conditioned desire for approval. Women are even more likely to give in to pressure to conform than men. In order to be at ease in a situation we need to feel accepted by the people around us. In hospital we are the junior members of a social group simply because we are on other people's home ground and not our own. Unless we follow their rules we will not be accepted. The labouring woman in hospital is caught between the Scylla of aiming to please and being accepted into a social group, and the Charybdis of following her own instincts and doing as her body tells her. Man being the highest social animal, the chances are that being accepted into the social group will take precedence over following one's bodily instincts. But these two instincts are at war with each other. Stress is the inevitable result of a mental conflict. Stress leads to difficult labour, to intervention, to lack of control, to more stress. A vicious circle.

Pressures to perform

Childbirth is the most dramatic performance of a woman's life. But it is a performance that is done best without a continual stream of actual and implied criticism. Medically controlled childbirth is like turning an everyday drive into a driving test, and at any stage of the journey the woman knows that the examiner can force her to stop the car and take over. Fear of failure saps self-confidence which leads to stress hormone secretion which slows down labour which increases the fear of medical take-over which increases stress hormones. A vicious circle.

Western woman abandons the security of her nest when she needs it most – during labour – and places herself at the mercy of strangers in totally alien surroundings. Her stress hormone levels soar, labour slows down because ß-endorphin, the contraction-stopping hormone, competes with oestrogen and oxytocin, contraction-promoting hormones. Adrenaline is secreted every time a telephone rings or the foetal monitor bleeps. Adrenaline is secreted every time a stranger pops his head round the door to see how things are going. Adrenaline is secreted every time a routine procedure is carried out – routine for staff but not for the mother. When control of labour is taken out of the hands of the labourer and put in the hands of managers, stress is vastly increased because the labourer is no longer allowed to act on her own initiative and follow her instincts. Instincts are given to reduce stress, to restore the brain's equilibrium, to balance bodily needs to the environment. If we ignore our instincts we should expect to suffer pain.

Pain

Conflicting hormonal forces cause pain which is a signal from the body for pain-avoidance behaviour. Instead of using our pain-avoidance instincts, however, we are encouraged to take pain killers. The civilised solution to pain in childbirth is to add powerful drugs to the hormonal cocktail controlling childbirth. Mothers taking heroin during pregnancy are loudly condemned but how many women realise that pethidine is a close relation of heroin and, moreover, that pethidine slows down uterine contractions? How many mothers know that epidural anaesthesia greatly increases the risk of a forceps delivery? Any drug removing the sensation of pain without removing the underlying cause will act against the instinctive control of labour making it harder and longer. Fathers are sometimes welcomed into labour wards only because often they can persuade the mother into taking drugs for pain she may not even feel and does not always want to obliterate. Modern woman needs the presence of a familiar person to help her to cope with an alien environment; and if that person is turned against her labour becomes yet more stressful.

On the other hand, women need the psychological support of their partners in hospital childbirth. One reason for falling mortality rates in recent years is that fathers have been encouraged to support their partners in labour. In one of the medical books there is a marvellous example of the psychological and hence physiological help a husband can give. Anecdotal though it is, it illustrates the point perfectly. A doctor quotes from a case where the woman was haemorrhaging before the birth of her child. He was desperately holding on to the uterus with both hands in an attempt to staunch the flow while the operating theatre was being prepared for a caesarean section; suddenly the woman's husband entered the room and the doctor felt the uterus squeeze his hand. The mere presence of a familiar loved figure affected the uterus (McLaren, 1961).

Hospital beds

On arrival at hospital patients are labelled, asked to change into nightwear and put to bed. All this confirms their child-like position in the hospital family. The medical dangers of going to bed have been known for decades but the habit persists. The late Dr Richard Asher outlined the dangers of putting patients to bed in his book *Talking Sense*, published in 1972. Tucked up in bed is the worst place for a labouring woman. She can so easily lose control of her own destiny; becoming a mere number, a case to be processed – Mr So-and-So's elective caesar in bed X.

Bed is normally associated with sex, sleep, illness and naughty children. Hospital beds are never associated with sex but always with illness. Hospital patients are often treated like naughty children and the use of beds in childbirth reinforces this idea. Childbirth is described by some as a sexual experience and no one would dream of having sex on a hospital bed, even fertility clinics instruct couples to have sex before attending the clinic and do not expect them to perform to order at the hospital.

Hospital is a place where people usually do things to you to make you better. Putting women to bed turns them into patients, the passive recipients of active professional management of labour. A hospital bed is not an appropriate place in which to labour from the psychological point of view. Neither is it appropriate from the physical viewpoint.

The professional attitude towards labouring women is seen all too clearly on the covers of their textbooks. At their best the book jackets depict a woman lying on her back and surrounded by medical gadgetry, with perhaps a nurse holding her hand; at their worst there is a cut-away picture of a uterus with a baby inside with the woman's face completely omitted. Books for the lay market have soppy pictures of women dressed in flowing white holding flowers – another distorted picture of maternity.

Technological Childbirth

And there is a new danger for modern women – technological childbirth. Western society is obsessed with science and technology, and medicine is no exception. All over the country groups of women and men are beavering away raising money for the very latest in childbirth and baby life support systems, foetal monitors and incubators. Modern man is no longer prepared to trust his own instincts but must needs measure, calculate and analyse his world and act on scientific observations rather than believe the evidence of his own senses. We have been brainwashed into thinking that science has the answer to all our problems.

I am not advocating a return to scientific illiteracy; my own work is founded on science. I am grateful to the scientists for providing the scientific evidence that stress does indeed interfere with labour. What I have found lacking is the human touch; relating findings to everyday life, to normal childbirth in normal women. The emphasis of most research is on pathology not normality.

There is a tendency to divorce science from everyday life – unless there is a profit to be made somewhere. There is no financial profit for manufacturers of specialised equipment and drugs in natural childbirth or home birth – nature herself provides the specialised equipment and the drugs. Scientific medicine

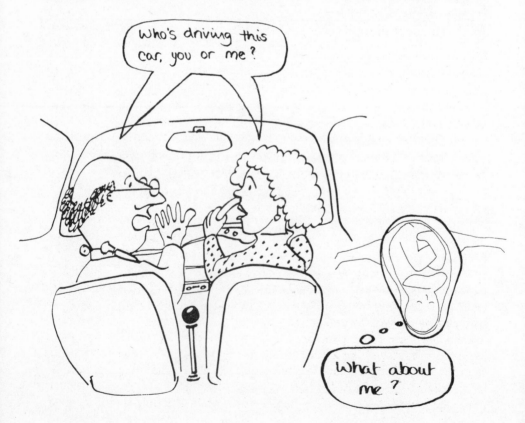

divorces the mind from the body; in their attempts to unravel what is going on in the uterus, the scientists forget that the womb is part of a human being. Today's scientists tend to fall into the twin traps of over-specialisation, and of allowing the love of pure knowledge to interfere with the true role of science, which must surely be to increase man's knowledge for the benefit of all. Virtually none of the very exciting work on stress hormones and labour has filtered down to the end user – the mother. The work on ß-endorphin has not even reached the obstetricians who might have been able to put two and two together. Neither has any of this research reached the midwives, not even the more radical of their number who have been waiting for scientific confirmation of their long-held suspicion that childbirth proceeds best in the absence of medical intervention. This is a timely reminder that we must not leave it up to the scientists to pass on their findings to humanity. They have different aims and have patently failed to see important implications of their work.

The science of obstetrics has manifestly failed to achieve the aim of improving childbirth for modern women. Death rates have gone down, owing to improved social conditions, but nearly all women are dissatisfied with the service at some level, even if only at feeling uneasy at the conveyor belt system.

There is a real sense in which medical childbirth creates physical problems for hospitals to cure. Surely there is enough ill health in old age requiring attention without having to create problems at the beginning of life as well? The remaining dangers of childbirth are largely caused by medicine itself. Even fear, the chief cause of stress in childbirth, is nurtured and sustained by the system.

Psychological stress of intervention

Hospital childbirth *per se* condemns us to hard labour but there is worse to come. Instead of removing the underlying causes of stress, the medical management of labour only serves to increase stress. Even the simplest measures which involve no physical interference whatsoever can cause stress, for example the labour chart, or partogram, which records the rate of cervical dilatation, comparing it to some artificial and arbitrary standard. Even Friedman, the obstetrician who invented it is reported to think that it may have caused more harm than good. The very measurement itself turns labour into a performance test, like the driving test. Merely recording the dilatation rate may cause a woman anxiety. If labour is progressing faster than average she will be reassured and labour will proceed well, but if she falls behind the standard 1 cm per hour, she will start to worry that something is going wrong, and, stress hormones having the effect they do, it is all too likely that something will go wrong. Foetal monitors are similarly unhelpful and have indeed been found to increase the number of forceps and caesarean deliveries without reducing perinatal mortality. Moreover they restrict movement, making the labouring woman less able to join in the dance of the foetus and uterus. Midwives listening to the foetal heart rate intermittently using Pinard stethoscopes, and recording uterine contractions by observation, do a far better job at monitoring labour than a piece of technology that restrains a woman's movement and physically invades her body. The benefit to hospitals of foetal monitors is one of cost, saving staff time – women and their partners become unpaid machine minders. Hospital horror stories contain accounts of partners rushing off to find staff when monitors emit terrifying flashes and bleeps, leaving the labouring mother on her own.

Vaginal examinations are intrinsically stressful; we are not used to our bodies being invaded by strange hands. There is simply no need for internal examinations to take place every hour on the hour.

Lucky indeed is the woman whose cervix dilates at or above the normal rate. Then she might be left in peace with her husband and a midwife for company and all may go well. But if she lags behind the norm, the cascade of intervention is set in motion and the odds on having a straightforward delivery become less and less.

Pain relief

At antenatal clinics, while still coming to terms with pregnancy itself, women are asked what form of pain relief they would prefer in labour. The unquestioned assumption that labour is painful is built into the system. Women are led to believe that labour will be painful and it becomes so. But contractions are not intrinsically painful and the pain of delivery itself is short lived. Certainly labour can become painful if it is not allowed to proceed naturally in stress-free surroundings, but pain is an instinctive signal to turn on pain-avoidance behaviour. For normal contractions nature provides a far better form of pain relief than any the pharmacist can devise. Artificial pain relief dulls the instincts and can actually interfere with the workings of the uterus.

Drugged mothers, dopey babies and hard labour

There is no safe drug for pain relief in labour. All analgesics cross the placenta and a dose high enough to give relief to the mother has a twenty-four fold effect on her baby, by reason of the disparity in size. Even seemingly innocuous drugs can have dire effects. *Aspirin* not only blocks contractions by inhibiting prostaglandin production but also makes the blood less likely to clot making post-partum haemorrhage more likely.

The dangers of *pethidine*, an artificial opiate, and thus a smooth muscle inhibitor, are too great to be contemplated from the point of view of both mother and baby. The mother needs to remain alert and able to respond to her instincts and thus control her own labour, and the baby needs to be fully alert and ready for its transition to life outside the womb. *Diamorphine (heroin)* is sometimes used to restart labours that stop on admission to hospital. It seems to relax women enough for normal labour to resume and the smooth muscle inhibiting activity does not seem to impede normal labour (see page 123). It seems that the artificial drugs similar to the natural endorphins and enkephalins have as widely varying actions in the body and brain as the endorphins themselves.

Sedatives and tranquillizers are often given instead of pain-relieving drugs for the specific purpose of making the labouring woman more tractable so that she will hand over control of labour to the professionals.

146

Epidural anaesthesia cuts off the nerve supply to the voluntary muscles needed for the second stage of labour, and delivery is often then achieved with forceps and an episiotomy, both of which will lead to real pain after birth when the mother needs all her strength to care for the new baby. The anaesthetic disrupts the baby's heat control system increasing the risk of heat stroke. Moreover, epidurals carry the small but not to be ignored risk of maternal paralysis. They also risk a dural tap, letting out some of the fluid (CSF) surrounding the spinal cord. This causes a headache for which there is no cure except time – the sufferer must spend up to a fortnight completely flat – not the best introduction to the joys of motherhood. This enforced immobility itself leads to a greater risk of deep vein thrombosis (DVT), a major blood vessel blocked by a blood clot, which can lead to life-threatening pulmonary embolism – a risk of all major surgery involving general anaesthesia.

The risk of thrombosis after *general anaesthesia* is well known and it should not be contemplated lightly for childbirth – newly delivered women are already at increased risk of thrombosis because their blood contains increased levels of a clotting factor, a natural response to oestrogen which evolved to reduce the risk of post-partum haemorrhage. The discomfort of contractions is as a pinprick compared to the pain of thrombosis, which feels like a night cramp and persists for hours. For breastfeeding mothers the treatment for thrombosis involves hospitalisation and self-injection of heparin three times a day for six weeks and this seems a high price to pay when one is also recovering from childbirth and caring for a newborn baby. These risks may appear small to staff but women must be told of the risks in order to be able to give informed consent.

Natural pain relief

I am not a masochist wishing to condemn labouring women to torture. Less invasive methods of pain relief exist for those who need it. Human touch itself is one of nature's methods of pain relief. Hurt children run to their mother for a cuddle, she will instinctively rub the painful place. Fathers are probably the most appropriate people to massage the pain away in childbirth but professionals could also cultivate a "hands-on" approach to pain relief. The environment for labour is important here; an uninhibiting atmosphere is needed for massage. There are various methods of stimulating the body's inbuilt pain-relieving mechanisms, among them transcutaneous nerve stimulation (TENS) and acupuncture. Hypnosis and meditation are also helpful and both need an atmosphere of peace and quiet.

Taboos

During the second stage of labour the negative influences of the strange hospital environment become yet more pronounced. Throughout our lives we are taught that sex and defecation are private matters. There is an enormous taboo on having sex in public and an even greater taboo on defecation in public. My three-year-old son sends me away after I have sat him on the lavatory because he knows he will not be able to perform even in the presence of his mother; taboos are probably innate as well as social. I have no doubt that even reading references to defecation in this book upsets the sensitivities of many readers. Yet the second stage of labour feels exactly like defecation – and our civilised society expects this event to take place in full view of complete strangers, some of them males, under bright lights, in a cold and clinical environment and, until recently, with the woman flat on her back with her legs strapped up in the air. Is it any wonder that so many babies end up being delivered by forceps? It is amazing that any woman manages to give birth at all in such circumstances. There is an appalling loss of dignity which puts a woman at a psychological disadvantage for the rest of her stay in hospital. Internal examinations are bad enough but can at least be passively endured; however, to expect a woman to push her baby out against all her innate and social instincts is little short of barbaric.

Woman have suffered this indignity for hundreds of years and countless numbers of mothers and babies may have died as a result. We will never overcome this taboo but can ameliorate the worst effects by warning pregnant women what to expect and by ensuring that the only people present in the delivery room are there by invitation. The labouring woman should know her midwife as a friend, and trust her in the most intimate way. The manner of professionals towards the women they are caring for is vitally important. If they have already become friends and are seen to be honest and trustworthy then unfamiliar procedures will cause much less stress. The very worse sort of intervention is carried out by professionals who fail to see the woman as a person and treat her as a case.

9   The Cascade of Intervention

". . . by getting away from Nature as we do, she hits back at us."

W.T.W. Nixon

The hormonal balance of labour is so critical to the efficient working of the uterus that any intervention, however seemingly trivial, is likely to upset it. The medical reasons for offering the intervention should be utterly compelling before any steps are taken at all. In the 1960s behavioural scientists researching stress responses to new situations found that the initial reaction of subjects to the first meeting with the researchers produced higher levels of cortisol (triggered by ACT hormone) than any other form of stress that could be devised. New situations automatically cause stress and any form of intervention involving unknown people and unknown procedures and equipment in a strange place must have a contraction-stopping effect on the uterus rather than a contraction-promoting effect.

Induction

On some day after the expected date of confinement (EDC) the obstetrician decides that induction is necessary to avoid the dangers to the foetus of postmaturity (the actual number of days post-term varies from obstetrician to obstetrician and from one to fourteen days). Some obstetricians are now questioning the need for induction, there is no danger to the foetus until the pregnancy has gone two weeks over term; but they are finding that women are now expecting to be induced soon after they become overdue and are indeed asking for induction – the effects of brainwashing of the 1970s persists. There is a 25% risk of caesarean section following medical induction, proof itself that induction is dangerous, and a very strong reason for doing it only when strictly necessary.

Drs O'Driscoll and Meagher have more to say on induction than most: "Induction extends the period of stress to which a woman is exposed by the time that elapses before labour begins... There is also a sharp increase in operative intervention... There is a sharp increase in the demand for pain relief." (*The Active Management of Labour*, 1986.)

Nowadays most inductions are for sound medical reasons, but having said that, I doubt whether many inductions take place at the weekend. The dangers to the foetus of remaining *in utero* for two extra days pale into insignificance beside the need to maintain an efficiently run maternity unit. It is my fervent hope that violent induction will become a thing of the past. Precipitating an infant into the world before his stress hormone system is mature enough to cope with life in the outside world is asking for trouble. There is always the possibility that dates have become muddled and the baby will face the dangers

149

of a premature birth needlessly. The chief dangers are respiratory distress syndrome and a relative lack of bonding hormones necessary for making the transition to a different way of life. The number of premature babies suffering from respiratory distress increased dramatically in the 1970s when the fashion for induction was at its height – I doubt whether many of the extra intensive care cots introduced as a result of this mismanagement have been decommissioned in recent years, I do not recall seeing any headlines announcing protests at cuts in the numbers of special care cots. And if the cots are there they will be filled.

It is likely that, for some women, the brain will continue to exercise its right of veto over the uterus and delay the onset of normal labour. We have been so brainwashed into expecting painful and dangerous labour over hundreds of years that it will take decades to reverse this widely felt fear. Some form of induction may still be helpful in years to come. I list the various forms of induction in ascending order of danger.

Education and reducing stress
Antenatal education to counteract learned fear of childbirth and measures to reduce stress at the end of pregnancy could reduce the incidence of postmaturity. Reducing stress at the end of pregnancy by providing home helps or giving the father the chance to take some of the burdens of everyday life from his partner's shoulders, for example by giving time off for household chores such as shopping and meeting the other children from school, could allow more women to go into labour naturally, which must always be the best option. Allowing women to give birth at home would help women with a fundamental loathing of hospitals.

Acupuncture
Acupuncture works by stimulating ß-endorphin pathways in the body. Many women have avoided having their waters broken (ARM) or invasive induction with drugs by having acupuncture. A woman threatened with induction could consider acupuncture as a gentle way of induction, bearing in mind that it sometimes takes a couple of days to work.

Cervical sweep
This is perhaps the least dangerous form of induction because it is only done when the cervix is ripe; but it is rarely used today. I suspect that this is because the timing of the onset of labour after a cervical sweep is unpredictable, varying between hours and days, and therefore the practice does not suit hospital routines. Midwives have known for decades that a fairly vigorous internal examination can trigger labour; a cervical sweep is one of the midwives' tricks of the trade. If the cervix is already softened and ready to dilate, then sweeping a finger round the cervix between the cervix and the membranes can trigger the onset of labour, perhaps by stimulating prostaglandin secretion or perhaps by stimulating pituitary oxytocin. If this procedure is carried out by a midwife known to the woman and sympathetic to the physical intrusion she is causing, it will not necessarily cause undue stress. There is no reason why this

procedure should not be done at home. Judiciously performed cervical sweeps could prevent transferring overdue women from low-risk, low-mortality GP units to high-risk, high-mortality consultant units.

Prostaglandin pessaries

Prostaglandin pessaries are used to ripen the cervix in the hope that labour will then start naturally. If the delay to the onset of labour is indeed caused by the vicious circle of a woman's stress hormones maintaining the block on the uterus which delays labour and causing yet more worry, then the knowledge that labour will start soon may be enough to trigger a normal labour. I see no reason why women should not insert the pessary themselves to avoid the stress of strange fingers in the vagina; most women are used to inserting tampons. They would thus take the responsibility for their induction if they thought it necessary and retain control. This procedure could be done easily at home.

Artificial rupture of the membranes (ARM)

Breaking the waters against the mother's will feels like legalised rape; I speak from experience. My obstetrician would not even wait for my husband (he was due to arrive in only five minutes' time) to perform this act of violation – perhaps he thought that my husband would side with me instead of him? I spent the next few minutes alone in floods of tears and was then precipitated into a violent labour, having to cope straight away with strong contractions for which I was totally unprepared, being a first-time mother. To add insult to injury the obstetrician had the impertinence to pop in after the baby was born to ask if I was happy about how it went. When I wrote to him afterwards to explain why I had responded somewhat rudely he did not even bother to reply – and obstetricians wonder why their insurance premiums are rocketing.

I doubt whether any woman knowing the possible consequences of ARM would ever give informed consent to this method of induction. (ARM in well-established labour belongs in a different category, see overleaf.) The advantage to the obstetrician is that he commits himself to delivering the child by whatever means that become necessary within the next few hours. The advantages to the mother are non-existent. Induction by ARM can lead to violent labour, for which the mother is mentally unprepared. The uterus is denied time to use the directive contractions of the first stage of labour to position the baby above the cervix; the baby suddenly experiences violent contractions for which it is totally unprepared, and these contractions may jam the cord against the uterus cutting off the foetal blood supply. The cord itself may become prolapsed, swept downwards with the flood of escaping amniotic fluid, putting the baby's life at risk. ARM may fail to work at all because a mother's uterus is simply not ready for labour, there may be far too few receptor sites for oxytocin to allow the uterus to function properly, labour will then be prolonged and tiring, calcium levels may be exhausted and lead to uterine inertia. Even if the uterus was ready for work, the baby is deprived of his protective cushion against stronger than normal uterine contractions for the last few hours of uterine life. The incidence of hypoxia (oxygen starvation) is far higher; more babies need resuscitation which is obviously a measure of an unhealthy beginning and which also leads to separation from the mother after birth. ARM induction brings a one in four risk of caesarean section – the very worst way of bringing a child into the world. ARM induction directly causes painful and dangerous labour. Contraction-promoting hormones and contraction-stopping hormones confront each other, each fighting to gain control; pain relief is hard to resist and there is no time to get used to the actions of the body and to learn how to cope with contractions. Instinctive control of labour flies out of the window until the mother manages to regain control of her labour which has so forcibly been wrested from her. Indeed she may never regain control and spend the rest of labour in a constant state of stress, probably ending up with the full cascade of intervention and deprived of her basic human right to deliver her own baby.

Of course, for many women, labour appears to start with the waters breaking, and it might therefore be argued that there should be little difference between the two types of labour; but there is all the difference in the world. Spontaneous membrane rupture may well be the first time the woman is *aware* of being in labour, but the onset of labour is notoriously hard to define and the hormonal bonds may already have been loosening for hours. The timing of membrane rupture is best left to nature, or at least to the midwife at the very end of the first stage when there is no longer any danger of cord prolapse.

ARM and Oxytocin Drip

Of all the methods of induction this is the most barbaric, and I choose the word with care. If breaking the waters fails to induce labour then it is an obvious indication that the uterus is not ready for labour, which very probably means that the baby is not ready to be born. However, by breaking the waters the obstetrician has committed himself to delivery within a specified number of hours. Throwing contraction-promoting hormones at a uterus not ready for labour is dangerous. The number of oxytocin receptors increases enormously throughout pregnancy, and even more during labour itself. An obstetrician has absolutely no way of knowing the hormonal receptor state of a particular uterus. Cases of uterine rupture and maternal death were not unknown in the early days of oxytocin therapy and the risk remains today. High artificial oxytocin in the first-stage may well result in changing the very nature of contractions by stimulating parts of the uterus other than those chosen by the baby.

Pain is virtually guaranteed – natural oxytocin comes packaged with met-enkephalin, a natural pain reliever that also dampens non-propagating uterine contractions (I suspect that the interference of A and B contractions causes pain). The woman is totally defenceless against the pain of unnatural contractions. She cannot change her position much because she is attached to a drip; she is probably also restrained by a foetal monitor which is seen as a mandatory adjunct to oxytocin induction because of the well-known dangers of induction. She has no option but to ask for pain relief which adds to the unpredictability of uterine action and her baby is often dragged protesting into the world by a pair of forceps or, eventually cut out of her protesting body to an uneasy reception in the neonatal care unit (paid for by the cash-starved NHS and charity).

Somehow we must dispel once and for all the fiction that modern, technological childbirth is safe and painfree.

Acceleration of Labour

Modern obstetricians are obsessed with timing; they equate a quick labour with a good labour, but many women prefer to labour in their own time and to avoid intervention. Nature has allowed a far wider margin of error in childbirth than the doctors' eight hours. The first stage of labour can go on for days and still result in a live birth, and yet some obstetricians are convinced that a rate of dilatation of anything less than 1 cm per hour is dangerous. Recent statistics have shown that the second stage of labour can last for up to four hours for first-time mothers, and two hours in subsequent births before it becomes dangerous (Tew, 1990). I am not advocating such time scales; I strongly believe that if we laboured as nature intended, the length of labour would be even less than the obstetricians' arbitrary limits.

Even today most women would prefer a more natural birth and instinctively feel that they do not want to rush the baby if it is not ready. However, they are not always given the chance to choose whether or not to have a particular procedure performed. For example the waters are still broken routinely in some hospitals, the implication being that informed consent is not necessary. Even when consent is asked women fear the consequences of refusing to sign. They know that they will be labelled as problem patients and treated accordingly, ignored and belittled. Patients need an almost super-human strength of mind to refuse hospital treatment, and even then court orders can be obtained to treat them against their will.

A woman whose labour has been accelerated must be monitored closely because of the increased risks involved. Many hospitals do not seem to have the staff to allow continuous monitoring by a midwife, particularly in the early stages of labour, and machines grossly restrict movement, leaving the woman unable to reduce pain by altering her position.

Established labour is often accelerated by breaking the waters or oxytocin infusion. Again breaking the waters increases the risk of cord prolapse and oxygen starvation for the foetus. It is also likely to lead to problems by preventing the uterus from steering the baby into the optimum position for the second stage. While still contained in his bag of waters the baby retains some freedom of movement but once the waters have been broken the mechanical dynamics of the uterus change. Violent contractions increase the need for pain relief and so further diminish the mother's self-control – increasing her ß-endorphin secretion. The cord is more easily constricted and the baby subjected to violent forces before he is ready. Again the baby may enter the cervix at the wrong angle and prolong the second stage of labour.

153

Prolonged second stage

Prevention is better than cure; women should be allowed to go into labour spontaneously and to labour at their own pace.

The second stage may be prolonged by a full bladder or a full rectum. A simple urinary catheter to empty the bladder may be all that is needed to enable a mother to deliver her child by her own efforts. As for a full rectum, nature intended the bowel to be emptied as the ß-endorphin block is gradually removed from the smooth muscle organs of the pelvis – but this does not happen in an induced or accelerated labour. The psychological stress of intervention increases ß-endorphin levels. Cultural taboos against defecating in bedpans within earshot of strangers do nothing to mitigate the problem.

Sometimes women are even asked to delay birth and wait for a delivery room to be prepared, or an obstetrician to arrive. I knew that this used to happen in the past, the American literature particularly is full of such horror stories, but I did not realise the practice persisted in London in 1992 until it happened to a friend of mine!

Episiotomies

An episiotomy is a cut made between the vagina and the rectum to widen the exit for the baby and to speed up the birth. Episiotomies were introduced without research because it was assumed that a man-made cut would heal more quickly than a natural tear and because doctors found it easier and quicker to sew up cuts than tears. Subsequent research has shown that tears heal better than cuts. Nevertheless, this form of intervention is proving hard to eradicate.

Prevention is better than cure. When birth is very close there is a great temptation for everyone, including the mother, to hasten it. Midwives are aware of this temptation and can help to prevent tears by encouraging the mother to "breathe" her baby out rather than forcibly ejecting him. A baby who is eased gently into the world will be less likely to tear his mother in the process. Episiotomies are also performed for forceps deliveries – but the perineum is designed to be stretched by the baby's head coming out rather than by a pair of obstetrical forceps going in.

In hospital, after the birth, the mother, still on the delivery table, waits for her episiotomy to be sewn up and yet another professional, or rather semi-professional, arrives on the scene – the junior hospital doctor. Young doctors learn how to sew on the delivery ward, and the consequences of gaining skill at surgical repair on perineums can be disastrous for a woman, her sex life and her marriage. I would vastly prefer to be sewn up by my GP who knows that he may see the effects of his handiwork in his surgery in the months to come or, better still, to be repaired by a woman, a midwife who is likely to have more respect for the perineum. In days gone by doctors were even taught to repair episiotomies with due regard to the male preference for a tight vagina during intercourse. The only way to avoid such physical assault is to avoid giving birth in a large hospital. Home birth, while not eliminating the risk of a torn perineum altogether, greatly reduces it and a botched repair is unlikely.

This is yet another area where the traditional skills of midwives are being eroded. Today, repairing tears is a separate skill taught to midwives on a special post-qualification course; if junior doctors get all the practice then midwives do not, and the need for a doctor in childbirth is perpetuated by lack of needlework skills on the part of midwives.

Forceps

Forceps are designed to pull, compress, and sometimes to rotate the baby's head to aid delivery. In days gone by doctors using forceps would brace themselves against the delivery table using the full leverage of their body to pull babies out, often with dire consequences for the child. In 1985 forceps were used for 10% of births in England and Wales and 50% of births in the United States. Before the advent of caesarean section forceps were the only way of delivering babies stuck in the birth canal.

There were three types of forceps deliveries depending on where the baby was stuck: high-forceps were performed when the baby did not descend through the cervix; mid-forceps were used in transverse arrest, when the baby failed to rotate to negotiate the bend in the birth canal; and low-forceps were used to pull the baby through the pelvic floor. High-forceps was very dangerous and has been universally replaced by caesarean section, and mid-forceps is a highly skilled manoeuvre now usually replaced by caesarean section. Low-forceps are still commonly used when the perineum refuses to stretch, but an episiotomy may well avoid a low-forceps delivery. Since episiotomies must be performed to allow the entry of forceps it might be as well to give a mother a little more time to deliver by herself after the cut has been made.

Babies are designed to be pushed out by the forces of the fundal muscle of the uterus and the mother's voluntary pushing. The head is designed to be compressed uniformly all round rather than between the two opposing blades of obstetric forceps. Delivering babies with man-made tools must be a treatment of last resort rather than a routine performance.

The risk of a forceps delivery in a teaching hospital is greatly increased because delivering babies by forceps requires considerable skill, and manual skills must be learnt by a process of trial and error. At present this skill is learned on live mothers and live babies. It should not be beyond the capabilities of medical technology to design a dummy baby in a dummy pelvis with simulated soft tissue for teaching students how to practice forceps deliveries. There is no doubt that forceps have saved the lives of many mothers and babies and that they will remain a useful tool for generations to come but they have been vastly over-used. Once again prevention is better than cure. I suspect that the need for forceps deliveries is greatly increased by denying mothers freedom of movement in the first stage of labour: the baby is far more likely to enter the birth canal at the wrong angle for an easy exit. Making mothers lie on their back for the second stage is similarly unhelpful; it is better to let gravity give a helping hand keeping the spine tucked out of the way, as it evolved so to do. I have yet to see any illustration of the second stage of labour in any book, professional or lay, when the mother was not lying on her back. The spine is always drawn nicely curved instead of flattened. My own body

155

"chose" a side lying position for me for the birth of my third baby. A hormone called relaxin is secreted which relaxes joints. A pregnant woman can dislocate her jaw by yawning. Relaxin enables the spine to relax a little at birth but if the mother is on her back it may well relax in the wrong direction.

Many forceps deliveries could be avoided altogether if doctors had a little more patience. There is no need to rush the second stage of labour and it is arguable that applying forceps to a baby already in distress will only add to his problems. The practice of rushing medical students in to observe difficult deliveries only compounds the problem for the mother who is finding it difficult to birth her child. If she were given a little more time with just a midwife and her partner for company she might well be able to push her baby out by herself.

Once again freedom of movement may help. And also furniture. The birthing stool is coming back into fashion because it enables a mother to use the strength of her arms and legs as well as her abdominal and pelvic muscles to help her baby out. A knotted sheet tied to the end of the bed was an old fashioned aid for mothers delivering at home. The more help a mother is given to push her baby out, the less will be the need for the baby to be pulled out by forceps.

Forceps were invented for use in the home and I see no reason why mothers in difficulties at home should be threatened with transfer to hospital for low-forceps deliveries. Surely it must be quicker for an obstetrician to drive to a mother's house with his instruments than to call an ambulance, transfer the mother to hospital, go through routine admission procedures and so on. The mother may even manage to deliver while he is on his way.

Elective caesarean section

I must admit that I cannot understand how anyone, knowing the facts, and in the absence of gross malformation of the birth passage, could possibly agree to deciding on caesarean section on a set date at the beginning of pregnancy. And yet, according to some obstetricians: "there are no contraindications to caesarean section". On the contrary, the only indications at the beginning of pregnancy for a mandatory caesarean section are a deformed pelvis owed to malnutrition, polio or rickets (which will vary according to the health of the population), or a physical obstruction such as an ovarian tumour (which has an incidence of 1 in 1,500). Only in such circumstances will the cost/benefit equation come out in favour of caesarean section. Even then it is vastly preferable to wait until the mother shows signs of going into labour naturally rather than to prevent natural labour by elective section two weeks before the expected date of delivery. Antenatal care is supposed to prevent problems in labour but actually *increases* the risk of operative delivery - relabelling more and more women as "high-risk" and transferring them to consultant care where operative deliveries become more and more likely.

Caesarean sections and cultural differences

The western medical model of childbirth fails women from many different racial and social cultures by trying to force everyone into a white middle class mould.

Language barriers and cultural taboos against male doctors in obstetrics only serve to make the situation worse. The further away from the middle class white ideal a mother is, the more threatened she may feel when required to labour in hospital, and the greater the risk that stress hormones will interfere with natural labour.

Asian women who often have a genetically small pelvis are particularly at risk of both elective and emergency caesarean sections. But this may cause them extra problems at home. They may be labelled failures by their husbands and their own community. But it is the NHS that has failed them by trying to force them into the hospital mould and failing to understand that different women have different needs.

If the medical profession wants to retain its controlling interest in childbirth it must start to recognise and cater for different needs. Yet it tried to bar the obstetrician Wendy Savage from practising altogether for doing just that. Home birth would seem a sensible solution to some of the extra problems arising out of cultural differences, it could cut across racial and cultural barriers at a stroke.

Inherent risks of caesareans

Despite modern techniques, caesarean section remains major abdominal surgery carrying all sorts of risks, not least the inherent risks of anaesthesia. The task of caring for a newborn baby while recovering from major surgery is horrendous. Certainly not a smooth transition to motherhood. Moreover, babies are designed to thrive on the stress of a vaginal delivery to prepare their lungs for fresh air. Mother and baby both need the stress of vaginal delivery to prime them for their first meeting. A mother who is delivered by caesarean section often finds it difficult to bond with her child. One study (Trowell, 1982) found that both one month and one year after birth, caesarean section delivered mothers maintained less eye contact with their children, and were more likely to lose their temper with the child. They reported "experiencing great problems with motherhood, confirming what difficulty they had in establishing a satisfactory relationship with their child". The incidence of postnatal depression is greatly increased; more surgically delivered mothers end up in a psychiatric hospital within three months of birth than do mothers following vaginal delivery.

The only possible psychological advantage, as far as the family is concerned, is that since the mother takes six weeks or even longer to recover from major surgery, fathers are forced to play a more active role in parenthood and so become more attached to their child. This apparent advantage is, however, overshadowed by the increased strain put on a marriage by the higher incidence of postnatal depression, problems with maternal bonding and prolonged stress of separation. Women are forced to remain in hospital longer following surgical delivery. What a price to pay for a closer relationship between the child and his father!

Ignoring the psychological outcome for mother and child seems to me to be a very short-sighted way of looking at childbirth. Elective caesarean section on a predetermined date must be the worst possible form of birth for mother, baby and family. Elective caesareans are often planned to take place two weeks before the expected date of delivery – that is when it is known that the foetal stress hormone system is immature. Surely there are enough premature babies without bringing more into the world? And for whose benefit is caesarean section performed?

Emergency caesarean section

The psychological effect on the mother of an unplanned caesarean section is predominantly one of failure. The old maxim for obstetrics used to be maintaining a position of watchful expectancy, assuming all was going well unless there was evidence to the contrary. In the days when caesarean section was physically even more dangerous than it is today, an obstetrician's competence was to some extent judged by his section rate. A good obstetrician had a low section rate and a bad obstetrician a high one. This is probably still an excellent way of sorting the wheat from the chaff when choosing an obstetrician.

These days an obstetrician may look somewhat embarrassed by a high rate but, as the operation is physically safer than once it was, it is more readily performed and, despite consumer resistance, is still escalating. There is now a new unwritten motto which reads: 'When in doubt, intervene'. It is this very intervention that is maintaining needlessly high levels of infant mortality.

Unfortunately modern technology is not as sophisticated as it is made out to be. Emergency caesareans are done in cases of foetal distress as measured by a foetal monitor but studies have shown that, while increasing the caesarean rates, foetal monitoring does not improve the success rate of live births. The usual reason for the absence of a foetal heart beat is that the baby has changed position and moved away from the sensor, but all too often the result is an emergency caesarean with all the consequent physical and psychological risks attached.

A leading obstetrician paints a grim picture of emergency caesarean section. His "purely imaginary" example is of a mother who smoked and drank during pregnancy, "had little antenatal care, although the midwife had been to see her three times" had planned a home birth and was admitted to hospital at 3 am on the day after the expected date of delivery with antepartum haemorrhage. The admissions team confirmed the problem and "phoned the obstetrician who gave his permission for the operation to proceed; he also added that he would come in *if it were absolutely necessary* [my italics]... A registrar at his lowest level of activity at four in the morning and an inexperienced anaesthetic registrar, together with an emergency night-time operating theatre team dealt with a lady whose life was already in danger and a baby whose life was teetering on the brink. They performed the operation, they gave her blood which somebody had to be called in to the laboratory to crossmatch. They... managed, by intelligent hard work, to save both the mother and her baby. This kind of emergency happens many times a month throughout the country. The risk of a mother dying following a caesarean section performed as an emergency, while small, is nevertheless four times that of the risk of dying or having a serious complication when the procedure is carried out electively." (Philipp, 1988, *Caesareans*, Sidgwick and Jackson). Emotive language is not confined to books on natural childbirth.

If this kind of emergency happens many times a month throughout the country why are the maternity services not better prepared for it? The home birth issue is irrelevant, the woman could just as well have been a woman planning a hospital delivery having had her full quota of antenatal care, and who gave up smoking and drinking while pregnant. The above quotation is a public and frank admission that *hospital services are managed to suit the staff not the patients*. Planned sections take place to suit staff and take place before the expected date of confinement when the foetal stress hormone system is immature.

The maternal mortality rate is now lower than ever before – but it could be lower still. Half maternal deaths follow caesarean section, and one in five of these follow elective caesarean section. Much more should be done to prevent the need for caesarean section in the first place. The caesarean section rate varies from about ten to twenty percent in NHS hospitals. Although some are indeed life-saving, most of these operations could be avoided altogether.

Indications and contraindications
Absolute indications for caesarean section are said to be transverse lie, cephalopelvic disproportion (too big a head to go through too small a hole), prolapsed cord and placenta praevia (where the placenta covers or partially covers the cervix) and heart disease.

Caesarians are also routinely performed for some older mothers, mothers who have had a previous section, foetal growth retardation and breech births; and emergency sections are performed for foetal distress, maternal exhaustion and prolonged labour. Test tube babies are also delivered by caesarean section in the mistaken belief that it is safer for the baby. Failed induction is yet another reason.

In Britain we are lucky that social reasons are no longer considered an acceptable indication for caesarean delivery; in the USA the section rate goes up to as much as 75% of all births in the days immediately preceding public holidays (Mitford, 1992). Elective caesareans are much more common in private medicine in the UK.

Of course planned caesareans will be safer than emergency caesareans as long as maternity hospitals are organised around normal office hours but unfortunately natural selection has not caught up with public holidays and a nine-to-five working day. Doctors wishing to find a specialty without unsocial hours would do better to choose dermatology – emergency admissions for skin complaints are very rare whereas, whatever the textbooks may say, women tend to go into labour at night. Emergency sections will always be needed for various reasons; and how much better it would be to review emergency procedures so that sections can be performed safely at all times – and to give all women the chance to go into labour spontaneously so that their child has the best possible chance of survival. The costs of manning efficient emergency services would be offset by decreased birth injuries and respiratory distress and lower maternal mortality. Potentially enormous savings could be made on intensive care cots and prolonged hospital stay for mothers.

Prevention is better than cure

The only completely unavoidable reason for caesarean section is placenta praevia. Nothing can be done to alter the position of the placenta itself. But placental position can be ascertained to some extent by ultrasound before labour starts. Women with low-lying placentas could be advised to go straight to hospital if labour starts with bleeding.

Previous caesarean

The old dictum "once a caesar always a caesar" is now discredited by virtually all obstetricians even in the USA. The risk of maternal death following a section is forty times the risk of death following the rupture of an old scar.

Disproportion

Disproportion is diagnosed when an obstetrician suspects that the baby's head may be too large to pass through the mother's pelvis. True cephalopelvic disproportion is rare in Western women; rickets and polio used to cause problems in deforming the pelvis, but these are diseases of the past. Mothers tend to produce babies to fit their pelvis. Disproportion may be diagnosed in error because it is very difficult to estimate the size of the baby even using ultrasound. Labouring mothers predict the size of their child with more accuracy than doctors using ultrasound.

Moreover, the joints of pregnant women are designed to give a little under pressure. Problems of babies becoming wedged in the pelvis are far more likely to be a consequence of the child entering the pelvis at the wrong angle, which is caused by denying women instinctive control of their movements during labour. If true disproportion is evident there is still no reason to plan an elective section on a particular date. It is better to wait for labour to start spontaneously and allow a trial of labour in hospital before intervening. At least the then foetal stress hormone system will be known to be mature.

Breech presentation and other malpresentations

Breech presentation is not an absolute indication for caesarean section. The birth is likely to be a little more difficult than a vertex (head first) presentation because the mechanics of the uterus will be slightly different – the head will not come first and exert an even force over the cervix, particularly if the waters have already been broken. Also the foetal head will not mould to fit the birth canal. As in other problems, prevention is better than cure. Breech babies can be turned in the weeks before labour in three ways: first through the simple expedient of asking the mother to kneel on all fours with her bottom raised for twenty minutes twice a day from about the thirty fourth week of pregnancy until the foetus has turned itself. This simple home remedy is successful in something like 95% of breech presentations. Second, acupuncture can be used to turn breech babies. Acupuncture works partly by stimulating ß-endorphin pathways in the body. ß-endorphin is intricately concerned with the mechanical action of the uterus in pregnancy and labour which gives a strong clue to the efficacy of acupuncture in turning breech babies. Third, babies can be turned manually from outside, external version. External version is no longer used since the manoeuvre is performed under general anaesthetic which carries the usual risks for mother and baby alike; and sometimes the baby would spontaneously revert to a breech position after the procedure. However, there is still no need to be told that a caesarean section will be necessary at an early stage of pregnancy – many babies turn themselves spontaneously into the vertex position before labour.

I suspect that many other malpresentations are better cured before labour starts. The medical textbooks show fearsome pictures of babies stuck in the birth canal with no visible means of exit, but I wonder how many of these are seen because mothers have been kept immobile during the first stage, denying the role of the uterus in tucking the baby into an oval position. Moreover, the foetal monitor, which is often the cause of immobility, is unable to give any information about foetal position. A "hands-on" approach to labour, where a midwife monitors the baby's position with her hands, would be infinitely preferable where malpresentation was suspected.

Again there is no reason why a woman should not be allowed to go into labour normally, so that at least one could be sure that the foetal stress hormone system was mature enough to stand the shock of caesarean section should it be needed.

Prolapsed cord
Prolapsed cord is an indication for an emergency caesarean but can itself be caused by amniotomy (ARM). It can happen in spontaneous rupture of the membranes which can take place anywhere.

Foetal growth retardation
It seems to me to be rather arrogant to "treat" slow growing foetuses by caesarean section. The assumption must be that a man-made incubator is better than nature's own incubator, the womb. High maternal and foetal stress hormones stop growth hormone secretion. How much better to relieve the pregnant woman of her stress; by allowing her partner time off work to help with the chores, or providing a home help. Dare I even suggest increasing maternity benefits to relieve financial stress in these hard times? If maternity benefits were reintroduced, vast savings in hospital costs could be made. Home visits by friendly midwives could be of infinite value in assessing the reasons for stress and giving practical advice and help.

Foetal distress, failed induction, maternal exhaustion and prolonged labour
Correct diagnosis of foetal distress is important. Foetal monitors do not seem to be very good at diagnosing foetal distress, and as some degree of foetal distress is a condition for normal labour at term, then it is difficult to find the dividing line between normal distress and life threatening distress. Failed induction, maternal exhaustion and prolonged labour are all indications of a poor understanding of the mechanics and hormonal regulation of labour. If

professionals knew as much about normal labour as they claim to know about abnormal labour the above indications for caesarean section would become virtually unknown.

Prevention and ultrasound

We should make technology our servant instead of our master. Various people have pointed out that ultrasound has been introduced with as little research as many other forms of foetal monitoring (Huntingford, 1984). I feel that here, just for once, technology is under-used. The benefits of pre-labour ultrasound could well outweigh the possible risks. Man has very probably adapted to ultrasound in his environment – we used to share our caves with bats. Ultrasound could be used at the thirty-ninth week of pregnancy to predict any problems likely to occur in labour, for example to determine the lie of the foetus and position of the placenta – to prepare the mother herself for potential problems and allow time for counselling should a caesarean section be proved necessary (thus preventing the need to obtain a court order for a caesarean section when the more usual methods of coercion had failed). At present hasty decisions are made in the middle of labour, after the predictable but unpredicted problem has already occurred and the mother is unable to make an informed decision about her treatment. It seems amazing to me that women still enter labour wards with undiagnosed breech presentation, transverse lie and placenta praevia. A woman knowing that the placenta was situated at the fundus could be better able to cope with labour knowing that it might be prolonged; forewarned is indeed forearmed. At present women have a routine scan at 16 weeks, mainly to confirm dates and to diagnose twins, but this information is of little use to her or her attendant in labour.

Hospital birth is intrinsically dangerous

Part of the reason for increased intervention is directly owed to the fact that 99% of births take place in hospital, and 95% of those in large, technological consultant maternity units. If the equipment is available it must be used to justify its existence or the departmental budget may be reduced.

The labouring woman is transformed into an object of scientific scrutiny. But the science of childbirth presented in this book has shown conclusively that, owing to the over-riding influence of the mind on the body, childbirth is an art, and an art practised by mothers and their mentors – midwives. The act of birth is, after all, the most fundamental of creative activities. Procreation may begin nine months before, but the foetus represents only potential independent life until it is presented to the world at birth. High-tech equipment is itself an admission of failure and should be hidden away out of sight. The very sight of such awesome gadgetry is enough to put a pregnant woman into a state of panic and send her stress hormone levels soaring. Yet all the latest technology is displayed with pride on pre-labour tours of the maternity hospital.

During labour the machinery becomes an alien barrier between the woman's mind and her body. The mere sight of it leads her to believe that something may go wrong and, the mind being what it is, belief can easily translate into reality. It is also a barrier between the labourer and her mentor. The role of a midwife is to be with women, to use her experience of labour to guide a mother into giving birth by herself. The machinery prevents the midwife from trusting her own senses. The modern midwife is being turned into a technician, a handmaiden at the beck and call of the doctor, the scientist. It is difficult to avoid contentious issues of feminism, and I cannot but wonder how this retrograde step has been allowed to happen.

After the Birth

Even after the birth the relentless hospital machine grinds on with more respect for management routines than for the new family. The hospitals have taken over the lying-in period as well as birth itself. Women are not deemed competent to deliver their own babies neither are they deemed competent to care for them. Indeed hospital birth often makes many mothers physically unable to care for their babies. After a caesarean section or with a dural tap headache a mother may not be able even to lift her baby out of his cot, let alone feed him. Even if both mother and baby manage to escape injury it takes even more effort to escape from hospital altogether.

My very real fear is that it may be too late to allow a swift return home to natural childbirth for the simple reason that there are no longer enough midwives who are experienced enough to trust their instinctive knowledge and do without the crutches of technology. The ultimate civilisation of childbirth is 100% medical control and, ironically, this could be contributing to the breakdown of civilisation itself by interfering in the next stage of the natural process – the bonding of mother and child.

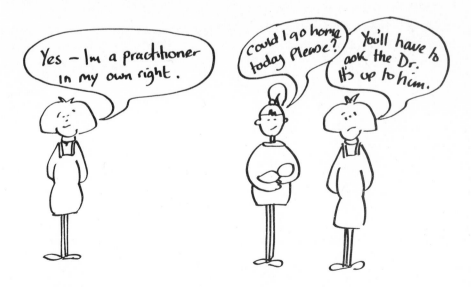

10 Bonding

Du lieber, lieber Engel du,
Du shauest mich an und lächelst dazu!
An meinem Herzen, an meiner Brust,
Du meine Wonne, du meine Lust!

(You beloved angel,
You look at me and smile!
In my heart and at my breast,
You are my joy and my delight.)

From *A Woman's Love and Life*, by Chamisso, set by Schumann

The time immediately following the birth is vitally important for establishing the relationships between mother and child, and within the family as a whole. The birth of the first child turns a legal marriage into a spiritual and biological marriage – the shared experience of that birth can provide far stronger bonds between man and wife than can the pen and paper of the registrar for births, marriages and deaths.

The birth of a child is also the start of a new family. No matter how many children belong to the established family, a new baby will elicit subtle, and less subtle changes in the interactions between all family members: the youngest child's position is now taken by the new baby and he may become jealous; other siblings who used to quarrel may join forces in an attempt to regain maternal attention; the father may have to look after the other children more than before. A new baby is always a shock to the family, which must change to accommodate the needs of the new member. A new baby will affect not only relationships within the nuclear family but also within the extended family – a mother-in-law may become a granny for the first time, a sister an aunt.

Parenthood can radically change one's total perspective on society and its institutions: childcare provision and education assume a new political importance; parents may become far more aware of long-term environmental issues as their temporal horizon extends to take account of their children. Life assumes a new meaning; parents live for their children's tomorrow instead of for their own today.

Parents have a totally new set of responsibilities to build into the existing framework of their lives; the attitude to life itself can change fundamentally, birth is an awesome experience for all involved in the process, but particularly for the first-time mother and her partner who now see their own genetic characteristics carried forward into the future by their child. Parenthood changes the position of men and women in society. Parents automatically become members of an exclusive club. Birth sets off a cascade of altered social connections which do not stop even with the extended family. For the moment, however, I will deal with the very first new relationship - mother and child.

Before the birth

There is already a relationship of sorts between mother and child dating from the first suspicion of pregnancy and enhanced at the time of quickening at about 16 to 18 weeks of gestation. The child is planned or unplanned, welcome, or resented. The child's behaviour in the womb will have given his mother ideas about his character which may bear no relation to his personality after birth. The progress of labour itself will affect maternal attitudes; an easy labour will tend to enhance positive feelings, a difficult or painful labour may reinforce negative feelings, but until the second stage of labour the foetus remains an integral part of its mother. He assumes a completely separate psychological independence from her only when he impinges directly onto the sympathetic nerves of her pelvis. For the duration of the second stage of labour the child is as yet unborn but has already assumed a separate psychological existence in his mother's eyes; other people will see him as an individual only after the birth of the head. When he is born the physical link between mother and child is also cut, and the child assumes ostensible physical independence.

Maternal behaviour

For the child to survive and develop normally a new physical link must be established and a new psychological relationship formed. The mother must respond to the child's physical and psychological needs and continue to nurture the child as much after the birth, by choice, as she was compelled to nurture him in utero. Psychologists refer to this process as bonding and have been studying its mechanisms since the Second World War. Natural selection has been perfecting the continuation of mother/child bonds over millions of years, and, again, one might reasonably expect evolution to have made a good job of the process.

In nature, the act of birth itself switches on a new set of behaviours for the mother – mothering. Stretching the vagina turns on prolactin, the grooming, nest-building and mothering hormone. Modern behavioural physiology textbooks state that human maternal behaviour is influenced more by culture than by physiology. If such is the case, then man has made a grave mistake in allowing culture to overrule nature. But all is not lost by any means. If we can allow culture to include knowledge of nature, as in labour itself, we can allow nature its proper place once more. Culture can teach mothers to obey their instincts instead of denying them.

Instinctive maternal behaviour is a combination of past experience and present biochemistry. Many studies, in animals such as Harlow's monkeys, and in man, have shown how parents' childhood experience influence their own parenting skills. Parents who were emotionally or physically abused in childhood are more likely to abuse their own children. If this sounds rather defeatist we must remember that, unlike Harlow's monkeys, man is better able to overcome detrimental effects of past experience through education.

Moreover, human society has a network of support groups and professionals which could be used to prevent such problems before birth instead of trying to pick up the pieces later on. A psychosocial profile of expectant mothers at antenatal clinics could prove as useful as a medical history. Another problem for us is that Western society gives young people scant opportunity for first-hand experience of childcare; families are becoming smaller and older siblings no longer gain experience through handling younger brothers and sisters. For many first-time parents the first baby they have ever held in their arms is their own child.

Bonding

Bonding is an interactive learning process between mother and child, starting at birth but continuing for months, if not years. Each teaches the other and each learns from the other. Maternal behaviour is designed to fulfil the child's physical and emotional needs. Before motherhood, instinctive behaviour is largely determined by personal needs; but now the helpless baby's needs must take priority. The baby is not quite so helpless as he may seem – he takes the first step in establishing a relationship. The behaviour of newborn babies is innate rather than learned by instinct. Already the baby knows how to search for the mother's breast and knows how to cry to attract attention. Already he can turn his head towards a noise and finds innate satisfaction in looking at human faces, particularly eyes, thereby eliciting a positive response from everyone he looks at. Most people find babies attractive – their relatively large heads and enormous eyes seem to be universally appealing. We all seem to be especially prone to appreciating miniature objects, and most women seem eager for the chance to hold a new baby and are delighted when the baby turns towards a breast that may have been dry for twenty years or more. By their very appearance and actions babies cry out to be mothered.

A baby is good at drawing attention to himself but his behavioural repertoire is very limited. Somehow he must teach his mother discrimination. He must learn how to tell her that he is tired, cold, uncomfortable, lonely, or frightened rather than merely hungry. His mother must learn his language before she can meet his needs effectively. Mother and child must gradually learn a new language together.

Mother and child must learn to communicate with each other and thus ensure that mutual needs are met. The more a mother and child understand each other's language, the better they will relate to each other. This first language is the precursor to all human relationships.

Relationships as shared language

A human relationship is a linguistic relationship, whether the language is verbal or non-verbal. As animal and primate, man has inherited body language capable of expressing a wide range of feelings. Man has the added advantages of speech and the written word. He has reached his present dominant position as highest of the animals by his vastly extended use of language.

We often speak of relationships between adults in the form of language. We get on well with people who "speak the same language" and feel barriers when our language differs from that of the person we are talking to. We cannot help but hear nuances of language which betray racial and social origins, level of education and even relative positions in professional hierarchies. We use language to define relationships and mark out territorial boundaries. Nearly all professions have exclusive vocabulary that distinguishes us from them and therefore maintains the professional/client relationship. However much we try to fight the tendency, we all use language cues to classify people on a continuum that runs from friend to foe. Language is used as much to divide people as to unite them. Even people who have suffered brain damage and are unable to understand the meaning of words know instinctively whether a speaker is telling the truth or lying by using body language cues.

The chief thing to note about language is that it takes a long time to learn – which is another reason for man's prolonged childhood. Language learning is an interactive process; it is a process of trial and error requiring constant feedback from the teacher reinforcing things that are right and correcting mistakes.

Physiology of language

There are various separate language centres in the brain that have evolved to enhance man's superiority as a communicator. We are born with innate mechanisms for learning and teaching language. We vary our language instinctively to suit circumstances. When adults talk to small children they raise the pitch of their voice, use short, well formed, simple sentences, talk slowly and use much repetition. The newborn baby is primed to listen to speech from the moment of birth. Chinese people find it extremely difficult to distinguish r from l because the Chinese language does not use the sound r, whereas English babies hear the difference between l and r within the first few days of life and learn that the two sounds are distinct. There are critical periods of language perception.

We use sight as well as sound to hear. People who are hard of hearing find it much easier to hear when they can see the speaker. The human face is infinitely expressive and we can tell meaning from facial expression even when we cannot hear the words spoken. Since the newborn baby is innately interested in the human face it is likely that his first communications will be facial expressions. The breastfeeding position is ideal for the baby to see his mother's face in perfect focus. Although babies tend to suckle with their eyes shut there are pauses in feeding when mother and baby look at each other and learn each other's facial language.

The First Meeting

Nature does not demand that we understand the subtleties of a baby's language at first attempt, but rather that, having fallen in love with our baby at first sight, we should develop the relationship throughout his childhood, supplying his changing physical and emotional needs until adulthood. The identical hormonal states of mother and baby following normal labour make them ideally suited to respond positively to each other without any need for language at all. After a natural labour, the newborn baby is in a highly receptive state of mind, fully alert and ready to perceive and learn about his totally new environment. His mother is in a very similar frame of mind, relieved that labour has finished and eager to meet her new child.

However, bonding is like any other romantic relationship, the initial euphoria of love at first sight must be replaced by stronger bonds if the relationship is to survive the test of time. Deeper attachments need time for the slow process of integrating the behaviour of each partner, so that the relationship becomes complementary and mutually satisfying. A developing friendship needs time for each to learn the other's language. People who have just fallen in love want to spend every second of every day alone together to cement the bond formed by the initial attraction. This is true also of the newborn baby and its mother and father.

Bonding hormones

The layman tends to assume that bonding is a purely psychological phenomenon but, as we have seen from previous chapters, it is impossible to split the mind from the body. After birth both mother and child have greatly increased levels of ß-endorphin which gives them a natural high and greatly enhances learning ability. Both have high levels of prolactin which switches on appropriate instinctive behaviour, which this time is not stress-relieving behaviour but instead stay-at-home and act-as-a-mother behaviour for the mother and nipple searching (rooting) activity in the baby. Prolactin release is also promoted by oxytocin, and oxytocin levels have been very high during the second stage of labour for the mother.

ß-endorphin thus continues its central role in childbirth after the baby is born by making both mother and child fully alert and ready to fall in love with each other at sight. Both are surprised by joy at the birth and see the world through rose-coloured spectacles.

Childbirth as a transcendental experience

A transcendental experience can be described as a vision of another world. People who have had such an experience report a feeling of eternity, or the certain knowledge of a better world; they report an overwhelming experience of peace; they report heightened awareness of light and colour. People speak of similar feelings following near death experiences; they see light at the end of a tunnel with loved ones waiting to welcome them to a better world – a world where they will be loved and cherished – the very experience of birth itself. Perhaps they are remembering their own birth. Transcendental experiences seem to be linked with ß-endorphin. ACT hormone and ß-endorphin are secreted as a result of all stressful situations, whether the stress is physical or psychological. People returning from clinical death report that in a split second they relived the major experiences in their lives, times when they were in a similar mental state, when ß-endorphin was also high, times of acute stress, whether pleasant or unpleasant. Transcendental experience often leads to profound changes in attitude to life. One marine who had a near death experience had to leave the army because he was no longer willing to kill.

Birth itself must be like a near death experience for the baby. After nine months of life in the womb, the foetus finds itself deprived of the protection of the amniotic fluid, squeezed through a narrow passage and forcibly ejected into a vastly different world. He is cut off from his oxygen supply and compelled to live in a totally new way. Birth is an enormous shock to the system; birth itself is the nearest most of us have had to experiencing death. The relief at starting to breath air and regaining physical contact with his mother must be enormous.

Childbirth is like a transcendental experience for the mother as well. The surge of ß-endorphin accompanying natural childbirth leads to a feeling of deep happiness, peace and joy. This feeling is associated with the child himself and provides strong motivation for mothering. Mothers are much blessed that nature gives them this profound life-changing experience to enable them to fall in love with their child. The ecstatic feeling gradually fades in the days following the birth but the memory of it remains.

ß-endorphin, then, is the physiological explanation for the bond that is made between mother and child when they are rejoined outside the womb.

Other roles for ß-endorphin

ß-endorphin has more mundane roles in addition to enhancing the joy of the first meeting. It also deadens any residual pain mother and child may have following the physical stress of birth. It enables each to imprint the other in their minds and it switches on instinctive behaviour by releasing prolactin. Babies given naloxone to counteract adverse effects of pethidine, an unnatural opiate, will be denied their quota of ß-endorphin, the natural opiate, and will therefore lose the enormous advantages it brings at birth and for the first few hours afterwards.

ß-endorphin is the hormonal mechanism for bonding, continuing the physical relationship of mother and child beyond the womb by enhancing emotional attachment.

There is already much evidence that the timing of mother/child bonding is crucial both for lower mammals, primates and for man. Shepherds know that they can persuade a newly delivered ewe to accept an orphan lamb if the lamb is presented by a certain time but that ewes will reject even their own lamb if the delay between birth and presentation is too long. Social scientists looking at human attachment have reported critical periods varying between one hour, twelve hours and three days. ß-endorphin secretion is highest at birth, the hormone remains active in the circulation for at least twelve hours which may account for two of the critical periods for bonding. Mothers seem to be given a natural high for about three days, post-baby blues usually start on about the fourth day, perhaps it is caused by withdrawal symptoms from ß-endorphin. Nature gives the mother and baby about three days to settle down with each other and gives them a kick start in learning each other's language by making them very receptive to each other. After this time the relationship is consolidated with the help of met-enkephalin, another endogenous opiate, released by breastfeeding. The nursing mother is given a psychological reward for feeding her baby which strengthens the bond.

Long-term attachment

The evidence appears to suggest that the timing of the first meeting is not the only important factor in developing attachment. The bonding process may start immediately after birth with mother and baby falling in love, but it continues throughout the lying-in period, and indeed throughout childhood. It is important to make the very best use of natural bonding hormones for the first few days of life. The more chances the mother and baby have to communicate with each other the better; the baby will learn to communicate his needs more quickly and the mother will learn how to relieve his distress sooner. This will lead to a settled baby, a happy mother and a peaceful life for the family as a whole. Language acquisition is a continual process, as the child grows and develops both physically and mentally his needs change. Normal development depends on the mother recognising and fulfilling those changing needs; it depends on good communication.

Physical Importance of Bonding

Health visitors and social workers are well aware of the failure-to-thrive syndrome where, despite apparent lack of physical disease, a child fails to grow and develop normally. Of course some children are genetically programmed to be smaller than others but this does not account for all the differences that are seen in practice. Poor communication between mother and child leads to poor growth and development of the child by two underlying mechanisms. First, the mother or caretaker is not very good at interpreting the child's requests for more food and so the child does not obtain enough to satisfy his physical needs; and second, because his needs are not being met, he has high levels of stress hormones which switch off growth hormone and cause retarded development.

A vicious circle is set up by poor language skills. If the child cannot communicate with his mother he must fall back on more instinctive behaviour. His repertoire of instinctive behaviour is very limited because he is so physically helpless. All he can do is cry, which tends to exacerbate the situation by reinforcing the mother's conviction that she is a bad mother because she is unable to fulfil her baby's needs and stop him crying. She interprets his cries of frustration as anger directed against her, becomes convinced that her baby does not love her and this leads to yet further delays in attachment.

In these circumstances both mother and baby can all too easily learn that they are unable to satisfy each other and both acquire learned helplessness which can have profound consequences to both mother and child. Learned helplessness was seen at its worst in Rumanian orphanages where the babies learned soon after birth that nothing they could do had any effect on what

171

happened to them. They became so docile, quiet and underdeveloped that the rest of the world was horrified. Children as old as seven were grossly underweight and apparently content to remain in cots with no facilities for play and only minimal care. Michel Odent has reported that African babies tend to achieve developmental goals earlier than Western children which suggests that their mothers are better at fulfilling their needs, both physically, despite higher poverty levels, and mentally. We are indeed lucky that most babies develop sufficiently and obtain their physical needs despite interference in the natural process.

A disturbed emotional relationship often becomes better once the child has learned to point or crawl to what he wants. Once he can do that, his body language becomes easier to understand, his mother is delighted that he can now communicate with her and the attachment process of mutual language learning can proceed more normally. But the roots of the relationship remain badly founded.

Hospital Childbirth and Attachment

The mother is not to blame for poor bonding. The absurdities of our Western hospital childbirth system destroy her maternal instincts before she has even started to be a mother. The professionals who refuse to believe that she can be a good mother without their help are the ones to blame.

More research has been done into maternal bonding in humans than in almost any other aspect of childrearing, but research in the social sciences tends to be scorned by pure scientists and by the medical profession who have a vested interest in defending current practice, and keeping hospital beds fully occupied. Bonding has become almost a dirty word for the professionals, perhaps because they have no way of measuring it. I find it very disturbing that a delay in mother/child bonding is now common enough to be considered normal, mothers are reassured that they should not expect to fall in love with their child at first sight, that it may take many weeks to develop an attachment. While this is undoubtedly true in this society, it is a damning indictment of hospitalised childbirth.

Mothers are lucky to be able to overcome most of the deficiencies of current childbirth practice, but many children are denied their natural birthright, and mothers are deprived of their natural maternal instincts. The hormonal control of labour is not merely concerned with getting a live baby out of a live mother but it is also a preparation for the new lives to be led by mother and baby.

The first relationship – A model for all future relationships

As long as we continue to see childbirth purely in terms of engineering and to deny the importance of bonding and attachment, we will continue to create social problems in the family and, ultimately, society as a whole. The first relationship is crucial for establishing man's humanity; it gives him a model for all other relationships in life and if we interfere with it, wittingly or unwittingly, we are condemning the child to a distorted perception of what it is to be human and to be part of society. Thus, the consequences of medical interference in childbirth go far beyond turning a natural event into a painful medical emergency - medical interference after birth disrupts society as a whole by interfering in the first social relationship and thus distorting all other relationships. Continued hospitalisation after childbirth can all too easily turn the first few months of family life into a nightmare. We are denying mothers and fathers the joys of parenting that should go hand in hand with the increased responsibilities that children bring. Even as I write another unforeseen possible consequence of poor bonding has emerged - *The Sunday Times* (May 17, 1992) reported that children given growth hormone to speed up their growth have been infected with mad cow disease - is this yet another hospital-induced illness that could be avoided by allowing mothers and babies the time they need together from the start of life?

Hospital practice
First-time mothers are advised to stay in hospital after the birth in order to recover from the ordeal of childbirth and to learn how to look after their baby. Natural childbirth is not an ordeal to be recovered from, it is rather a labour of love, hard work but infinitely rewarding. Hospital is such an intrinsically stressful place that it should be the last place in which to recover from any ordeal. Doctors are finding that people recover from the physical stress of surgery more quickly when they are treated as day patients or have only a short stay in hospital. But after birth healthy mothers and healthy babies remain in hospital under medical supervision, either from choice or as the result of emotional blackmail.

The New Patient

In hospital, as soon as the baby is born there is a new patient to deal with, and a new set of professionals spring into action and intrude on to the scene. The cord is cut straightaway (leaving enough to join on to blood transfusion equipment - just in case) and the baby labelled with a tag because, as soon as the physical link between mother and child is cut, there is always the possibility of muddling babies up, particularly in a busy unit with a nursery. The baby's airways are nearly always cleared by suction, whether needed or not - a precautionary measure. The child's weight, head circumference and length are recorded - in this scientific age we seem to need to measure everything that can be measured. The child is cleaned, gift-wrapped in hospital clothing and presented to his mother, now wearing his numbered label, his gift tag. There has already been a delay to the first meeting of mother and child; already the child belongs to the hospital; the hospital has made a present of the baby to the mother and this is proclaimed loud and clear by the label until the mother and child are allowed home when it can be removed at last.

The hospital is *in loco parentis* for the child - and also for the mother. The mother is treated like a child who is not able to take responsibility for herself and certainly not adult enough to take responsibility for her own child. She is

173

under enormous psychological pressure to do as she is told, she is in foreign territory and subject to pressure from authority figures. Staff have subtle ways of disciplining mothers who refuse to conform, the easiest of which is simply to ignore or belittle her in front of other staff and patients. She must be taught how to be a good mother, how to feed, change and bathe her baby. Only then will she be allowed home – and a professional eye must be kept upon her until day 10. Even then the baby is not discharged to the mother's care – but to the care of a health visitor. Society's authority over the child is firmly established from the moment of birth. Right from the start the mother's confidence in her maternal instincts is eroded and she is taught that she is irresponsible. Responsibility belongs to the NHS acting for the state. Is it really any wonder that parents are taking the state at its word and blaming teachers and the police, representatives of the state, for the increase in vandalism and anti-social behaviour? Medical childbirth teaches us from the outset that children belong to the state and the state is responsible for them. This is yet another self-fulfilling prophecy.

Time to share

After the birth mother, father and baby need time to "fall in love" and get to know each other, but unfortunately time is in short supply for hospital staff, although it hangs heavily on patients. Instead of leaving the new family in peace, the conveyor belt process must continue until the mother is settled into the postnatal ward. Each move to a different place entails more mental energy wasted in coming to terms with different surroundings and new staff – energy that would be better spent in bonding with the baby.

Paradoxically, a torn perineum may thus be a blessing in disguise to the family, to be exploited to the full. The family can remain where they are until a junior doctor is located and comes to repair the damage. The father is usually allowed to hold the baby while the mother is being repaired. The sooner he does so, the sooner he will realise that babies are not as frail as they appear, and the sooner he will start to form a relationship with his child. It is not only the mother who needs to bond with her child. However, all too soon the mother is put to bed in the postnatal ward, with instructions to stay there for four hours for fear of post-partum haemorrhage, she is unable even to lift the child from its cot and must wait for staff to hand her the baby when it suits them. The father is sent back home to enable his partner to rest.

Thus far I have considered only the scenario following a normal delivery in hospital when little pain relief has been needed. The situation following a forceps delivery or a caesarean is far worse. For the mother the joy of achievement that follows a spontaneous vaginal delivery is lost, she feels a failure and blames herself already for not being a good enough mother, not realising that operative deliveries are nearly always the result of a failure of the system rather than the mother's inadequacy. Add to this depressing scene the effects of the pain itself of a difficult labour and the drugs given to ameliorate it. The reasons why the mother feels unable instantly to bond with her child become even plainer. The mother sees her child as having caused her suffering and already feels a certain ambivalence towards him instead of joy at the first meeting. She is still feeling whoozy with drugs and her movement is greatly restricted; she may not be able to cuddle her baby, let alone feed him – she must wait until the pain-relieving drugs have been eliminated from her circulation. If the baby has been delivered by caesarean section she may not even be conscious of having given birth at all and the baby that is eventually presented to her might belong to anyone. The mother has not received her natural doses of ß-endorphin and prolactin. Caesarean section deprives her of natural learning and mothering hormones. One baby in six is born by caesarean section in the UK and the proportion in the USA, where operative deliveries pay better than normal deliveries, is far higher.

Neonatal intensive care

If the mother is lucky she will be able to keep her child with her as she is wheeled to the recovery room; the delivery room will be needed for the woman behind her on the baby production line. The mother is transferred to yet another new place, with another group of professionals to meet. If she is unlucky the child will be sent to the neonatal special care unit. Parkinson's law comes into operation at this stage – work expands to fit the available space. If the neonatal care unit has surplus capacity, then babies will be found to fill it. Hospital politics come into play again – use it or lose it – keep the neonatal care cots full or they will be cut and the department will lose status. Neonatal care units have undoubtedly saved many babies from death but how many babies have been deprived of their mothers at this most crucial stage of life simply because there were cots going spare?

Do fragile babies need incubators at all? One doctor working in an African hospital, where there were none, found that the mother herself made a perfect incubator – warm, soft, food on tap, the ever present comfort of the familiar heartbeat. This doctor saved 90% of babies as small as 4 lb. Contrast this with the well-established research findings that mothers of babies spending time in neonatal care units find it more difficult to bond with their babies, suffer more postnatal depression, are still talking to their babies less a year later, and are more likely to batter those children.

Medicalised childbirth itself fills the intensive care cots by creating damaged babies: for example, babies born with respiratory distress syndrome caused by premature induction; caesarean babies denied the positive benefits of the stress of vaginal birth; babies starved of oxygen during birth by unnecessarily hard labour and overstrong oxytocin-induced contractions; babies born floppy (a medical euphemism describing the rag-doll-like forms of babies requiring resuscitation) and full of artificial drugs. Babies deprived of the stress of normal birth are also deprived of ß-endorphin needed to fall in love with their mother and learn their new environment. When the mother has had pethidine late in labour the baby is given naloxone to counteract the effects of the drug – but this counteracts his own ß-endorphin at the same time. Depriving these children of their mother is adding insult to injury.

Think also of the likely affect on the baby of the clinical surroundings of an incubator. The journey from the security of the uterus to an intensive care cot is likely to have been traumatic in itself, but the ultimate transfer to a completely artificial environment devoid of human touch cannot fail to have lifelong effects on the child. If the first prolonged impression of the world is one of machinery, flashing lights, loneliness and isolation then what hope of a peaceful life can there be? Much more research is needed into the effects of care in the first few days of life. Neonatal intensive care must be the policy of last resort and certainly not the "just in case" attitude that prevails in high-tech hospitals when there are spare cots.

Psychological Costs

Babies born in hospital see the hospital as their first home. They will get used to hospital life only to go home when they are a few days old and settle into a new environment all over again. The return from hospital is a notoriously difficult time for parents and baby; if it can be achieved while mother and baby are still high on ß-endorphin then the transition may be less painful, but how much better to avoid the transfer in the first place by giving birth at home. Hospital is the very worst place for parents to start to learn their child's language. It can be compared to trying to learn a language from scratch by sitting in a busy airport departure lounge, waiting for one's plane to be called. There is too much background noise, too much stress, too many other languages being heard.

The mother has to learn to distinguish her baby's cry from that of twenty other babies. Patients have to learn hospital rules and routines, many of which are unwritten and must be worked out by a process of trial and error. In large hospitals a different set of staff work on the postnatal ward. In alien places people are quite simply under too much stress to learn anything useful; they must learn the new environment and the new people before they can divert attention to anything else. The mother must make her first attempts at caring for her baby under the scrutiny of strangers, many of whom give her conflicting advice according to their differing perceptions of good practice.

Consider also who must do the learning and what is to be learned. Both mother and father need to learn their new child's language and he must learn theirs; yet the father is largely ignored by the hospital after the birth. As a visitor he has a lower status than the mother herself and feels ill at ease, being a male in a largely female environment. Neither mother, father nor baby need to learn much about hospitals and how to cope with the stresses they impose; neither mother nor baby need to get to know people who they will never see again in their lives; neither should waste their energies learning the unwritten rules, the hospital routines. The hospital environment is totally artificial and bears no resemblance to home. All that continued hospitalisation achieves is to delay the time when the mother and child learn how to relate to each other in the surroundings and routines of everyday life – at home.

Spending a few days in hospital after the birth interferes with the process of transforming love at first sight into a more permanent bond. At home, visiting midwives can provide more than enough babycare instruction, and that

176

instruction is tailored to the home where the child is to be brought up; tailored to the individual needs of individual mothers, babies and families.

Large institutions require rules and regulations for efficient functioning and hospitals are no exception. Maternity units are less regulated than once they were, market pressure has allowed women a greater say in how they wish their babies to be treated, but in the end the hospital has the final word about everything. Professionals are legally responsible for patients under their care and can overrule mothers' wishes in all circumstances. Hospital routines are in direct conflict with the real need of the mother and baby which is to spend time together in peace in order to get to know each other, to learn each other's language.

Although rooming-in is now recommended practice, crying babies are still taken away from their mothers to avoid distressing other patients and to give mothers rest. One of the most important things for a new mother to learn is how to stop her baby crying, and the only way to do that is to experiment with various strategies until she finds one that works. A crying baby is communicating a need for some sort of attention; he is a learning opportunity for the mother or father. If professionals take over too readily the mother is denied this opportunity. It is useless for her to learn that someone else is better at calming her baby, not only will she miss her aides when she returns home but her lack of confidence is reinforced. Nearly all crying babies can be comforted by the breast but constant nursing is frowned upon for the sake of the mother's nipples.

The hidden message
Rather than teaching mothers competence in childcare, the opposite is taught – hospitals tell women that they need to stay in hospital in order to learn how to look after their own baby. The hospital's hidden message is that all first-time mothers are incompetent and, for many reasons, this may become a self-fulfilling prophecy. Just as in labour, the less interference by medical management in the mother/child relationship the better. It has long been acknowledged that mothers wanting to establish breastfeeding are better off at home, the let-down reflex ejecting milk is inhibited by stress. The more people there are who try to teach the clinical management of breastfeeding the less likely they are to succeed. New mothers need support and advice from one trusted friend, a midwife who knows the problems and has helpful hints up her sleeve. A constant stream of different people trying out different methods learnt from textbooks is counter productive. Breastfeeding is a very personal activity and not suited to the hospital environment when one never knows who will pop his head round the door next. Constantly weighing the child before and after each feed is probably the best way to promote bottle feeding. Babies are designed to lose weight for the first week of life; the mother's milk does not even come in until the third day. Newborn babies are stronger than we think, some babies buried in the rubble caused by the Peruvian earthquake survived for six days with no care at all.

The consumer society

Much of the instruction in hospitals seems to be related to learning how to use consumer products - the newly delivered mother is showered with free gifts, bounty bags, in order to turn her into a good consumer of baby products and so fuel the baby goods market. The much praised free market economy is not so free after all, it is distorted in all sorts of ways, one of which is by giving freebies to mothers in hospital. Some of these products may even be dangerous - recently, talcum powder has been implicated in childhood respiratory problems.

Proprietary baby food is very expensive for what it is, in May 1991; baby rice cost nearly ten times as much as adult rice (84p for 100g for babies; 98p for 1,000g adult rice). Even so, in March 1992 the price tag of a leading high street chemist's brand of baby rice had risen by 40% to £1.25 in less than a year. Prams and pushchairs have become high fashion goods, with colours changing each season. They are manufactured using non-removable unwashable fabric in pastel shades designed to date and age quickly thus deterring resale in the second-hand market. The price of a standard type of pushchair tripled between 1986 and 1991. The price of a pushchair parasol sold by a leading high street chemist doubled between 1986 and 1989. New mothers are a captive market, made all the more captive by bounty bags, and a market where guilt factors are played upon to the full - good mothers use X, Y, Z, the implication being that bad mothers do not. Most products are used for only a short period of time so mothers do not notice huge price increases. Parents of young children are taken for a ride by the big companies who seem to charge what they think the market will stand rather than pricing goods according to the relationship between raw materials and production costs. I suppose that it is naive to think that baby food should be less prone to market forces than other goods but it seems a pity deliberately to increase the cost of living in vulnerable groups such as families with young children.

Costs to society

I think it no statistical coincidence that the divorce rate is reaching record levels. Hospitalisation after childbirth teaches husbands that they are not needed and that childcare is women's work. If more babies were born at home, husbands would be able to bond with their children sooner and share responsibility for the baby right from the start. If the first few days are spent in hospital, men feel excluded. They look forward to the homecoming but the first few days are very stressful; the husband expects his wife to return home knowing all about babycare and thinks that life can then go on much as usual, but once home the baby seems like a different being. His routine has been upset, he has to sleep in his own cot in his own clothes. There are no longer neonatal nurses to help at night; and his mother is constantly worrying whether or not she is feeding him right. Perhaps her own mother has come to stay to help with the new baby - bringing with her conflicting advice she learnt from Dr Spock twenty-five years ago. The health visitor calls with yet more conflicting babycare doctrine. It is not surprising that mothers get frustrated, angry and tired and that their husbands are only too eager to return to work (if they have managed to obtain leave at all). Women resent being stuck at home all the more and family life becomes a burden for all; divorce is the easiest option. More and more women are choosing to be single mothers because they see the stresses married women experience as being even greater than the demands of single parenthood.

Lying-in At Home

Home is the best place in which to learn how to be a good mother. There are no hospital routines, no visiting hours – the father can help as much as he likes and the mother can spend time with her other children reassuring them that the new baby does not lessen her love for them. Family routines are less disrupted. There is no need for constant hospital visits. No baby-sitters are need for the husband to make partners-only visits in the evenings. There are no professionals closely watching every move. There is no competition with other mothers, no comparisons to be made. The community midwife comes to the home as a welcome visitor providing reassurance that all is well rather than trying to teach babycare. The GP pops in to meet his newest patient.

Even though a newly-delivered mother is not at her peak of physical fitness, with aches and pains in all sorts of peculiar places, she is likely to be up and about sooner and to recover more quickly. Some help will be needed around the house, particularly in helping to look after the other children and in shopping but the need is not as great as it was in the days before disposable nappies, automatic washing machines and tumble dryers. It will do no harm for the rest of the family to make do with microwave meals instead of home cooking for a few days. The family can adapt slowly to their new life and enjoy their baby in peace and quiet. Some extra help would be welcomed and women having a home birth are still eligible for home helps; although now the service is means tested.

Families Need Fathers

In our society "women's work" is still despised and denigrated – by women themselves as well as by men. Childbirth is an ideal opportunity for mothers and fathers to start to share domestic responsibilities more evenly. Women can be as reluctant to let their men loose in the kitchen, or to trust them with the vagaries of the washing machine as men are to take over. Childbirth forces women to ask for more practical support and their partners to supply it. Paternity leave is as important as maternity leave in the making of a new family. The father needs to bond with his new child and the child with his father. Parenthood should be a joint responsibility. Assigning men simply to the role of money-maker is as short-sighted as chaining women to the home. Paternity leave should not be seen as an optional extra but as a means of laying the foundations for happy family life and a more equal society. Children need a closer relationship with their father to gain a different perspective on the world.

And they need a mother who has a break from childcare once in a while for her own personal development. A mother chained to her children for twenty-four hours a day can become all too easily bitter and resentful.

Long-term effects

Man is a social animal. His first social relationship is with his mother. If this relationship is disrupted right at the start of life it may well lead to antisocial behaviour in later life. Like the writer of Proverbs in the Bible, I believe that disciplining children, teaching them right from wrong, and not yielding to the child's every whim, is part of parental love. A good parent will teach his child that he cannot always get his own way. After all, when he grows up he will soon have to learn to accept society's rules. Lack of parental discipline has been blamed for very many problems in our society. The subject crops up time and time again on Radio 4's *Any Questions*. Each time there is a split in the panel answering the question. Those on the political left blame society while those on the right tend to blame the parents. Perhaps left and right can now unite and blame lack of parental discipline for society's ills while at the same time blaming society for its gross interference with birth and mothering. Perhaps I go too far. I hope to research into this aspect of the hospitalisation of birth myself. All the physiological and hormonal research I have done has been merely a preamble. What really interests me about the psychology of childbirth is the effects on the family and society as a whole.

The spoilt brat syndrome in America has been explained as the direct result of medicalised childbirth and consequent lack of bonding between mother and child – but it keeps the wheels of commerce whirling round. Unable to feel the normal rush of maternal feelings following a hard labour ending in a difficult delivery, the mother feels guilty that she does not love her baby enough. She covers up her ambivalence by providing physical proof to society that she is a good mother in the way that Western society recognises best – she buys presents. The present buying continues throughout childhood, the child is given all that he asks for at the drop of a hat. His every wish is granted. There is a whole generation of children who have never had 'no' said to them; who think that money provides the answer to life's problems. Unfortunately spoilt children grow up and eventually learn that life is not such a bed of roses. Is the soaring crime rate in the UK and abroad a direct result of spoilt children continuing to act as if the world was there for the asking?

11 Politics

"There is a holy mistaken zeal in politics as well as in religion. By persuading others, we convince ourselves"

Junius (18th century frustrater of knavish tricks)

First of all, it is important to explode the commonly held myth that choice in childbirth is just a women's issue, and a feminist issue at that. The way we bring our children into the world affects the whole of society, not only women. Labelling the issues as purely feminist skates over the rights of both the father and the child, both of whom have a legitimate interest in childbirth; assigning issues in childbirth to the political fringe ignores its importance to the rest of society.

It is all too easy to see childbirth merely as a feminist issue because childbirth happens only to women, but women's issues are the province of all women whether or not they would call themselves feminists. Superficially at least there is a power struggle between predominantly male obstetricians backed by a patriarchal Government on the one hand, and exclusively female mothers backed by predominantly female midwives on the other. However, this analysis of the problem is too simplistic. Women are not the only people concerned with childbirth, fathers have feelings about birth too and so do male GPs; neither are all obstetricians ranged alongside the Government. There are two separate struggles going on at the same time. There is a struggle between midwives and obstetricians to decide which of two professional groups should manage normal childbirth and there is a struggle between ordinary people and the system itself. Most mothers are not interested in professional politics – they talk in terms of fighting the hospital system, and that system includes the midwives themselves.

The politics of childbirth concerns far greater struggles than that of the feminists: it epitomises struggles between man and machine; between the individual and bureaucracy; between intuition and reason; and between art and science. These struggles are between the individual and the machine, whether it be the bureaucratic machinery of society or the physical machinery of technology. Bureaucracy and machines are often described as faceless, and both treat those they deal with as if they also had no face, as if their human needs and feelings were of no importance. The politics of childbirth can be thought of as struggles for control between mothers, midwives, obstetricians, health service managers and the State. Who wins the struggle depends on who has the most power. Childbirth politics is power politics. It is indeed a fight between weak woman and strong man but it is also a struggle between trade unions – between the Royal College of Obstetricians and Gynaecologists and the Royal College of Midwives, and it is a struggle between midwives themselves, the more conservative midwives who have bowed to medical pressure and let doctors take over the control of normal childbirth, and the Association of Radical Midwives who are fighting to retain professional autonomy in the face of opposition from all quarters.

Territory

Childbirth politics concern territorial rights. The three usual places of labour fall into territories controlled by three different groups. Home is obviously the territory of the parents. Despite their name, GP units are primarily the territory of midwives because in reality, although capable of overruling midwives, GPs bow to midwives as the true experts in labour (any GP unwilling to do this would be unlikely to take on women for GP unit delivery). Consultant units are the territory of doctors. Doctors specialise in disease in all other medical specialties – including gynaecology which is so strongly linked with obstetrics; it is therefore natural for them to see childbirth as a pathological, disease-ridden process.

The history of the maternity services has been one primarily of the gradual encroachment of specialist doctors into normal birth, the territory previously controlled by parents and midwives, so much so that the very role of the midwife herself as an expert in normal childbirth has been successively eroded until we reach the situation where, in Eire and the USA, she is actually relabelled a maternity nurse. This encroachment reflects the insidious reclassification of childbirth as a disease to be cured rather than a normal life event. It reflects the current medical opinion that labour can be viewed as normal only in retrospect.

The term obstetrics is of relatively recent origin. Thirty years ago obstetricians considered themselves artists and their own textbooks included the term midwifery in the title, but many modern obstetricians would feel insulted to be termed practitioners of midwifery. The terms themselves reflect the contrasting views of labour. "Midwife" is an old English word meaning "one who is with women" and "obstetrician" comes from Latin and means "one who stands before". Doctors practising meddlesome midwifery used to be condemned by their colleagues, but now labour is actively managed on behalf of a passive patient.

The obstetrician as surgeon
Obstetrics is a surgical discipline. Doctors becoming members of the Royal College of Obstetricians and Gynaecologists call themselves "Mr" again to mark their inclusion in the ranks of Master Surgeons. Surgeons solve problems with the knife. Physicians retain the label doctor: they solve problems without recourse to surgery and call in a surgeon only when they have failed to treat the patient as a whole person.

By concentrating on physical barriers of bone, muscle and soft tissue in childbirth, obstetricians fail to recognise hormonal and psychological barriers which can be removed with less injury to body and mind. They remain sceptical about anything they cannot see, feel or cut into. They tend to welcome technology that can visualise or measure what they cannot see. The surgeons rushed to embrace ultrasound and the foetal monitor without bothering to conduct clinical trials. The surgeons like concrete data and are reluctant to admit that the midwives' and GP physician's "hands-on" approach could be more appropriate for childbirth.

Surgeons have a higher status both in the hospital hierarchy and society in general. This is probably owed to the fact that their efforts are immediately tangible and visible. There is a certain kudos surrounding surgical patients that is not shared by people going into hospital for other reasons. Surgery has inherent risks and nursing care must be more intense to counterbalance the trauma of bodily invasion, giving people the illusion that more has been done for them. Surgery is seen as the ultimate in hospital care and people can even feel proud that they were ill enough to deserve such special treatment. Surgery is usually the most expensive form of treatment in terms of both equipment and staffing costs, and a society measuring worth by money spent sees it as the ultimate in care. Surgery is also far more dramatic and gives people the chance to be the centre of attention for a little while. However, a new mother and her baby are naturally the centre of attention in the family at least and can well do without the added attention of the surgeon's knife.

Surgeons have a different attitude to their patients. In surgery, the split between body and mind is translated into reality. Surgeons cannot operate on the mind and so they are tempted to ignore it completely, seeing their patients only as bodies. They can all too easily forget that their patients are able to talk and may know something about their own body that the surgeon does not know. This can easily lead to ridiculous mistakes. A surgeon instructed to remove a cyst from my neck removed a mole instead, a waste of his time, my time and NHS money. The surgeon's natural inclination is to intervene, the physician's is to forestall surgical intervention.

Recent advances in *in vitro* fertilisation, surgical intervention at the beginning of foetal life, have given obstetricians even more kudos, but in fact IVF is as nothing compared to the miracle of fertilisation, pregnancy and birth wrought by nature herself. The adulation of surgery today probably represents an enormous cost to society, money which could be far better spent improving the living standards and consequently the health of those at the bottom of the heap, those who are least likely to seek and receive medical help even when medicine could improve their lot. It goes without saying that surgery takes place in hospitals. Hospital is the territory of the doctor/surgeon/scientist and the natural home of medical technology. Dr Vernon Coleman has much more to say on this subject in his book *The Health Scandal*.

Consultants versus GPs

Each professional group is fighting to preserve its territory against further erosion and, at the moment, stalemate has been reached. Obstetricians have attained 95% control; midwives, with the aid of GPs, retain 5% control. Midwives have retained their control only with the help of GPs; without continued GP acceptance of midwives' expertise the last GP unit would have been closed years ago. The fight is as much between general practitioners and hospital consultants as it is between midwives and obstetricians. The place of the GP as an independent practitioner outside the hospital services has been crucial in retaining the right of women to have their babies at home. There were not enough maternity beds to allow all women to deliver in hospital until after the 1960s baby boom so GPs practising in the 1960s and before had experience in home deliveries. After the baby boom obstetricians needed to keep the beds full in order to keep their jobs. They have managed to do this ever since but there were always some GPs convinced that hospital is not necessarily the best place in which to deliver babies.

As these older doctors retired there was a real risk that home birth would be outlawed. Junior doctors learn their obstetrics in large teaching hospitals with state of the art technology, a tiny minority of trainee GPs have the chance to see a home birth. They are rushed in to see complicated labours, and later on in their training junior doctors are only called by midwives when something goes wrong. They simply do not see normal labours, so they come away with a grossly distorted view of childbirth.

Even sympathetic GPs can deter women from a home confinement by the words "If you had seen what I have seen [in hospital] then you would not even consider it." What doctors have seen is determined by their pathology oriented training. However, education itself is changing. Instead of blindly accepting all that is taught students are now taught to question accepted wisdom and one result of this is that a new generation of GPs offering home births is emerging. These GPs are still young and the GP is nearly at the bottom of the medical hierarchy. A young GP is still risking his professional career in allowing his patients home deliveries, but he has less to lose than his hospital colleagues – in deciding to become a GP he was not aiming at a consultant's post anyway.

Medical students
Medical students spend about six weeks on maternity wards and each has to deliver several babies before qualifying. One student was reported by Susan Spindler in *The Times* thus:

"You feel very gauche walking up to a person you've never met before and saying at a very intimate point, 'Come on, push this baby out, really try hard.' And when the woman is in pain you don't really know where to put yourself."

This student said that he became emotionally inured to childbirth. One wonders whether he had any idea of when a woman should push, how to prevent a torn perineum, and how to deal with his own embarrassment, let alone her emotional needs.

If our babies are not actually delivered by a student, they are delivered by doctors trained to become hardened to childbirth.

Midwives
Midwives have been pressed into the service of the State since the time of

Moses when they had to report births of male Jews in Egypt under the Pharaohs.

Being so closely concerned with life and, in the past, death, they have been greatly feared by both the Church and the medical profession, both of which have taken pains to reduce their power. Witches (largely female midwives and healers) are no longer burned at the stake but attempts are still made to excommunicate midwives and female obstetricians refusing to toe the party line. Modern midwives have been put firmly in their place by the medical profession as a whole, and it will strongly resist all attempts to return power to midwives and the women they serve.

The oldest and most natural profession of midwifery has been reduced to subservience to a male dominated view of birth – a glorification of science and technology to the exclusion of humanity and common sense.

Management

The NHS is a vast machine that has resisted all attempts to find an acceptable form of self-management. As for maternity hospitals, they are quite simply too big. Expensive technology has been concentrated in large maternity hospitals as a way of maximising its use in an effort to reduce overall costs, but herding large numbers of labouring women into hospitals creates other problems, not the least of which is that women feel depersonalised. It is deemed impossible to organise large scale services and at the same time provide continuity of care and to treat women as individuals. The midwives who staff the antenatal clinics are not the same ones who deliver babies or who cover the postnatal wards. The logistics of providing women with a named midwife to care for them throughout pregnancy, labour and postnatally are seen to be too horrendous to contemplate. It is indeed impossible while the present shift system for midwives remains but if the shift system were changed it would be possible.

There are pockets of humanity within the machinery of the system itself. After all, even bureaucratic machines are made up of individual human beings. But when individuals are governed by rules and regulations, and risk losing their jobs if they step out of line, then there is little scope for individual variation of anything other than bedside manner. It is as hard for a staff member to treat each new woman she sees as an individual as it is for the woman to come to terms with seeing so many different people in the course of pregnancy, labour and postnatal care.

In isolated GP units and at home it is possible to treat women as individuals, but access to technology is limited in these places and technology is seen as more important than continuity of care. Technology has thus replaced human observation in the maternity services as the main route of maternal monitoring. Indeed scientific measurement of all processes in childbearing has become a necessity. When a woman is seen by different people at each antenatal visit, and where her labour overlaps more than one shift, then observations must be written down in a scientific way to enable the next member of staff in the chain to get an impression of progress. It must be nearly as stressful for midwives working in large amorphous hospitals as it is for women delivering there. Obstetrics by the rule-book is as damaging for midwives as it is for their patients.

The only person who is likely to be seen more than once during pregnancy is the consultant himself but he is unlikely even to deliver the baby, let alone spend time with his patients during labour. He is far too busy overseeing all the other women in his care. He manages labour at a distance by a set of rules and regulations to be followed by staff who work under him. Different obstetricians in the same hospital may have different protocols to manage labour, sometimes midwives have to look at the notes to see which obstetrician is named in order to know which set of rules to follow.

Technology – The New Religion

We have fallen in love with technology while at the same time we worry that it is taking us over. The scientist still thinks that his thinking is based on solid fact unbiased by political and personal opinions. However, his thinking is no less biased than mine. Science is no more than a collection of working hypotheses all based on the experience of the world as we know it. As our experience of the world is infinitely varied so are the hypotheses we form in an attempt to make sense of experience. Arguments between scientists become heated as their viewpoints vary. The hypothesis of the role of stress in labour presented in this book is just another hypothesis but it does attempt to take account of the role of the mind in the workings of the body.

Science and technology have become an obsession, and medicine is the route by which most ordinary people come into contact with modern science at a personal level. Medicine, with its emphasis on cure rather than care, is thus seen as the embodiment of all that is good with modern science and technology. The doctor has replaced the witch doctor and priest of the old order, a role for which he is unfitted by the preponderance of science in the medical curriculum with its emphasis on factual knowledge. We are taught to believe and trust in the modern wonders of science to such an extent that some of us are all the more prone to react with court action when it does not cure our ills, although most of us still tend to think that doctors are infallible. We still do not realise that much of medicine is still based on informed guesswork rather than scientific fact. The doctor/scientist has feet of clay, he has been built up into a modern magician but his subject is that most complex system, the human body, about which there is far more unknown than known.

Much of the doctor's time is spent dealing with spiritual problems translated by the body into physical problems and the doctor is still taught primarily to cure only the physical manifestations of mental unease leaving the primary cause of disease unrecognised. The mystique of medicine has replaced the myths of religion in the role of curing man's ills but it does not pretend to deal with his soul. At least the witch doctor was concerned equally with body and soul. Replacing religion with science and technology leaves man's soul unattended.

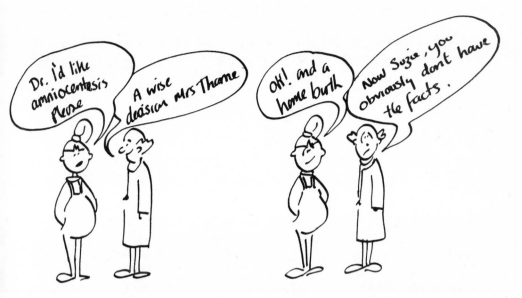

Hospitals have become new temples to the glory of science and technology, full of mystical equipment understood only by those in the inner circles. Mere mortals, mothers and fathers, must defer to the high priests; the temple maidens, the midwives, must wear the uniforms of temple servants, while the doctors don the white robes of priestly purity. Pregnant mothers are easily identified by their maternity wear but sometimes fathers must respectfully remove their jackets on pre-labour tours to pay proper respect to the new gods.

Delivery rooms are the anterooms to the Holy of Holies – the operating theatre. Lower mortals may peep round the door of delivery rooms during pre-labour visits but are allowed in only a few times in their lives. The operating theatre itself is forbidden in all but exceptional circumstances. This is the age of the scientist doctor cocooned in his superior knowledge and attendant technology, protected from his patients by an entourage of go-betweens.

The technology of childbirth is operated by human beings, regulated by other human beings, but all too often the machine tenders are required to suspend belief in their own observations and rely on the machine itself instead, thus placing the mind of the machine above the mind of the operator and reinforcing the tendency to watch the machine rather than the mother – as if the machine rather than the mother was having the baby! The operator does not even need to be in the same room as the mother – foetal monitors can relay information on the baby's heart rate and mother's contractions directly to a nursing station. In a very real sense machines are replacing midwives, and no wonder the midwives are fighting their corner. No wonder labouring women feel like battery hens. In the face of such mechanisation, no amount of communication skills and psychological input into training will convince me at least that the trend towards increased technology is anything but retrograde.

187

Childbirth and the State

The State did not start to get unduly concerned with childbirth until the scientific age of the mid 19th Century. The State had an interest in maintaining population levels to man the factories and ensure a mass market, and to man the army to protect trade interests abroad. These issues are predominantly monied middle class issues. The middle class entrepreneurs needed people from whom to make their fortune, people both to manufacture and to buy their products. Having made their fortunes they sent their sons to school to learn how to become gentlemen and to brush off the aura of trade from their personages. The father had not made enough money to finance them all in the manner to which they had become accustomed so some sons became the new professionals – doctors and scientists while perhaps the family purse could be stretched far enough to allow another to become an MP. These were the men who solved problems by throwing bricks at them – building hospitals, hospitals that were to provide business contracts for the father and scientific material (patients) for his son. They were not, however, good enough for his wife and daughters. His womenfolk were not to make a mass exodus to hospital for another fifty years; they continued to have their babies at home. This was also the age of invention – the Victorians were notorious for inventing and selling gadgets of all sorts. Here began the love affair with technology and here lie the roots of our modern way of birth.

By the 1940s, the drug industry had cured the worst danger of hospital childbirth, puerperal fever, by the invention of antibiotics and now hospitals were "safe" for middle class women as well as working class women. Advances in anaesthesia were made. Hospital childbirth seemed even more attractive in wartime when the population was more mobile and husbands were away and unable to help with domestic chores. It seems almost unbelievable today, but just after the Second World War there was considerable concern that the birth rate was falling below replacement level. Pregnant women were cherished as never before and given maternity beds in hospital. The maternity services never looked back. There was no need; maternal and infant mortality were falling fast and increased hospitalisation was the obvious cause.

The greatly feared decrease in population did not in fact occur but by then the bureaucratic and technological machinery was in place, the obstetricians were trained and needed posts, and women went to hospitals to have their babies in ever increasing numbers to provide training material for students and patients for the consultants.

Since the inception of the Welfare State, the State also has an interest in reducing the numbers of unhealthy children born that would otherwise be a drain on its resources. The doctors' lobby in Parliament is quite strong enough to convince the government that the services are imperative to prevent birth mishaps. There are very few women MPs of childbearing age. Female Conservative MPs tend not to trust the average woman to choose what is best for her baby, and female Labour MPs tend to fight for improved hospital services out of habit. Maternity services are the one area where the government is still quite happy to spend vast amounts of money while not requiring audited accounts.

Official government policy is still that every woman should labour in surroundings that have access to the latest technology in case something goes wrong.

Paradoxes in the NHS
Community care
The biggest paradox in the NHS maternity services is that elsewhere the trend is towards community care. Geriatric hospitals and mental institutions are being closed and the former occupants returned to the community. Community care is thus seen as appropriate for people with mental illness and the diseases of old age, but the community is no longer strong enough to support these people, it falls to a small number of people, usually women, to provide the support that used to be offered by the wider community in the pre-Victorian era.

It is unquestionably a fact that nearly all pregnant women are healthy and yet they are still herded into hospital for birth. Obstetricians are still aiming at 100% specialist unit deliveries although it has been obvious for some time that they will not achieve that goal.

Consumer-led demand
The present government is in favour of using the market forces of consumer demand to determine services provided. In the health services it is the GP rather than the patient who is the consumer. The GP has a budget to choose hospital services for his patients and NHS Trust hospitals provide services in relation to local demand from GPs. As usual market forces are distorted by advertising, NHS Trust hospitals are spending £25 million a year creating artificial markets. Hospitals are spending vast amounts of money on buildings and technology to make it politically unacceptable to close hospitals no longer needed.

In the maternity services choice is severely restricted by GPs themselves, who may refuse to offer home or GP unit delivery, and by the hospital services available. Women have virtually no choice in how or where to labour. Most women are offered a choice between one or two high-tech hospitals rather than a choice between a high-tech birth and a low-tech birth. Some hospitals offer low-tech birth rooms but these are not always available when a woman arrives at a hospital in labour. Moreover, these rooms remain within the context of high-tech consultant units, under the ultimate control of the medical staff, and some midwives are reluctant to use them. It is still up to the obstetrician as to how much choice a woman can choose to exercise.

GP units still exist but tend to exercise strict controls over who is allowed to use them, for example first-time mothers under 30, other mothers under 35, those delivering between 37 and 42 weeks of gestation, women taller than 5'6". There are numerous occasions for booking instructions to be changed throughout pregnancy and the maxim appears to be "if in doubt, transfer to consultant care." In one study of a GP unit, of 1585 women originally booked

189

for GP unit delivery, only 1267 (80%) laboured there, and of these 9% were transferred to consultant care during labour or after delivery. The perinatal mortality rate was very low at 4.7 per thousand. According to one obstetrician critical of GP unit care, who failed to give mortality rates for a similar cohort of women under his own care, "... on paper this seems to be an excellent result." (Philipp, 1989). Not only on paper but in reality this is an excellent result. It is a result that could be repeated up and down the country if GPs and midwives were allowed to regain control of childbirth.

Cost effectiveness

Hospital childbirth is not cheap: it requires much manpower, from the ward orderly to the obstetrician, paediatrician and anaesthetist; it requires expensive drugs; it requires expensive technology from foetal monitors to well-equipped operating theatres and neonatal intensive care units; it requires enormous buildings which are expensive both to manage and to maintain. If, as some authorities now maintain, hospital childbirth is not even safe, then the State is spending an enormous amount of money perpetuating a system which may actually damage mothers and babies adding to medical and social costs. Home birth is cheap, the mother feeds and houses herself and her baby. Instead of an expensive obstetrician she needs a midwife and a GP, who is paid just £25 for his services. GP units are comparatively cheap since they dispense with the services of specialist doctors and do not need purpose-built specialist buildings and high-tech equipment.

Personal responsibility for health

Health education gained ground in the 1980s, campaigns designed to promote public awareness about how to keep healthy – "Look after your Heart" and the anti AIDS safer sex message were presented loud and clear. "Prevention is better than cure" summarises the argument *against* hospital childbirth in a nutshell. The specialists maintain that modern practices prevent obstetric disasters but this book shows that problems in labour can be prevented by freedom from interference itself. If women were encouraged to take as much personal responsibility for childbirth as they are for giving up smoking and alcohol for pregnancy, then many problems in labour would be prevented.

Waiting lists

In the NHS the waiting list is the major form of rationing. Access to hospital services depends more on availability of beds and staff to cover them than anything else. In recent years other forms of rationing have been developed as demand has outstripped supply but the maternity services is the only branch of hospital services that manages to do without a waiting list – for obvious reasons. Rationing by waiting list ensures that, money and staff permitting, services are fully used all the time. If there is no waiting list in obstetrics it must mean that the services are underused at least some of the time. There are only a few ways to maximise use of maternity facilities. The main way to do this is to use facilities when they are not actually needed. Expensive equipment can be justified by the number of patients using it. If not enough patients benefit in reality this fact can be obscured by using it on women who do not need it. This involves turning low-risk patients into high-risk patients and the consequence has been that more and more pregnancies are defined as abnormal and requiring sophisticated care. Relabelling low-risk patients as high-risk is yet another self-fulfilling prophecy.

The Winterton Report

The State has a justifiable interest in the maternity services. Taxpayers foot the bill for the services themselves and, directly or indirectly, for the costs of mismanagement of labour, through damages paid for birth mishaps, or through the health and education services which care for disabled children and adults. Obstetric practice has far-reaching economic effects on society as a whole, and it is right that the State should have an interest in maternity services. MPs represent taxpayers in parliament but have little say themselves in how the country should be governed. Power of government is vested in only a small proportion of MPs. The government sets up select committees to enquire into areas of interest and there have been various such committees in the past dealing with maternity services. Until 1992, the recommendations of these committees have always been to transfer more and more responsibility to hospitals and consultant obstetricians but, in 1992, the House of Commons' Health Service Select Committee chaired by Nicholas Winterton, produced an astonishing report. It recommended that women should be given more choice over where to have their babies and more control over the kind of care they received – including epidurals, caesareans and inductions. The report stated: "We believe that the debate about place of birth, and the triumph of the hospital-centred argument, have led to the imposition of a philosophy of maternity care which has tended to regard all pregnancies as potential disasters, and to impose a medical model for their management which has adverse consequences on the way we think about maternity care... There is no convincing and compelling evidence that hospitals give a better guarantee of the safety of the majority of mothers and babies. It is possible, but not proven, that the contrary may be the case." (*The Times*, March 5th, 1992).

Maternity care is not a feminist issue – this committee was chaired by a male; a Conservative MP, one of the least likely people to have an interest in feminist politics. The present Minister of Health is a woman and one would have thought that in the present parlous state of the economy nothing would now stand in the way of full implementation of the report's recommendations, which include the following

- *We recommend that the policy of closing small rural maternity hospitals on presumptive grounds of safety be abandoned forthwith*
- *We recommend that the development of midwifery managed units, combined with effective continuity of midwife care between the community and the hospital, should be pursued by all District Health Authorities*
- *We recommend that the Department of Health take steps to impress*

upon all GPs their duty to facilitate the wishes of women, especially in respect of their choice of place of birth and their right to midwife only care

- We recommend that it be a duty placed upon GP practices to have in place arrangements for women to have a home confinement with GP cover or midwife only cover if they so desire
- We recommend that all maternity services be obliged to publish figures relating to operative intervention and stillbirth and neonatal mortality rates over the previous five years, and to make these figures available to women booking with that service
- Above all, it [the committee] requires an affirmation that the needs of mothers and babies are placed at the centre, from which it follows that the maternity services must be fashioned around them and not the other way round.

The science of childbirth as exposed in this book is in full agreement of all of these recommendations, which seem more than reasonable even without knowing the role of stress hormones in labour. But we have yet to see any signs at all that the recommendations will be acted upon.

The government still tacitly assumes hospital to be safer (Command Paper, July 1992):

- We remain convinced that the safety of mother and child is of overriding importance... It is impossible to predict all the problems which may arise in labour... most births take place in... hospitals because of the ready availability of emergency facilities in case something goes wrong... We now have the lowest ever levels of perinatal and infant mortality. Maternal deaths are thankfully very rare... Advances in technology have played a significant part in this achievement.
- existing arrangements already offer considerable flexibility for women to be given a choice in the type of maternity care they receive... Health Authorities... need... to accommodate wishes as far as possible, within local policies and resources [Who determines local policies and resources? Managers and consultants with a vested interest in keeping their jobs]
- A desirable feature in the process of care is that a woman should be cared for by the same group of professionals throughout. [Thus the concept of a named midwife has been replaced by "the same group of professionals"]
- We are convinced that there is a role in the maternity care of each woman for each of the professional groups, who, by working in a partnership within which there is an agreed leader at each stage, can provide a "seamless" pattern of good care. [Unless the agreed leader is a named midwife or even the woman herself, this recommends maintaining the status quo, where the leader is the obstetrician.]

The Losers

In all this the baby has no voice at all, he is completely helpless, he is at the mercy of all the rest. Because he cannot speak for himself, others speak for him. No doubt everyone believes that they have the best interests of the baby at heart, so much so that the mother often feels that she is little more than an incubator. Since birth is more dangerous for the baby than the mother (far more babies die at birth than mothers die in labour) the physical needs of the baby are automatically put above the physical and psychological needs of the mother and she feels even more powerless. A dangerous legal precedent was set in October 1992 when a court overruled a mother's decision not to have a caesarean section. According to a barrister specialising in medical cases the decision is important because:

"It establishes that although the mother was competent to refuse the operation, her absolute right to decide treatment could be overridden in this case, on the ground that the operation might save the child's life, and would do no harm to the mother."

The doctor's clinical freedom has been extended even further and now transcends the human rights of the mother (*The Times*, October 14th, 1992).

The other losers are the midwives, fathers, family life and, ultimately, society itself. A society that lets technology take control over such a fundamental aspect of life, the birth of its children, is fast leading to a society where technology is more important than humanity.

Obstetricians, backed by the full force of the law, seem to be the winners but they themselves have become little more than the slaves of technology. But in this society the slaves of technology have more status than the servants of humanity - mothers, midwives, priests and teachers. Consultants rule the NHS and the maternity wards, their clinical freedom is now protected by the courts. By virtue of their status and power they determine government policy for the maternity services and the voices of mothers and their unborn children are crying in the wilderness.

12 Flat Earth Science

"It is the folly of the world, constantly, which confounds its wisdom."

Oliver Wendell Holmes (1809-1894)

In general it is true to say that scientific thought is still being stifled by the constraints of verbal and symbolic reasoning. Common sense and intuition is thought to have no place in medical science unless it can be backed up by hard facts. But even hard facts can stare doctors in the face to no avail. It takes many years even for research based on hard facts to filter its way down to clinical practice. Moreover, doctors decide which hard facts they are going to take notice of and which they will reject out of hand. The history of medicine is full of tales of scientific breakthroughs in knowledge followed by years and years of failure to act on research findings.

Contrary to popular opinion, no matter how many hard facts support research findings, no scientific theory can ever be proved conclusively. A hypothesis is merely a theory that fits the facts as they are known at present. *The hypothesis that hospital birth is safer than home birth does not even fit the statistical hard facts* and yet it is proving well nigh impossible to dislodge from medical thinking and teaching.

Some theories fit so many available facts that we regard them as fully proved. It was once believed that the world was flat. A flat earth fitted everyday experience so well that it was unthinkable that anyone could see it as a sphere. But different people have different viewpoints. First the astronomers started to look at the available evidence for a round earth and then Magellan circumnavigated the globe, and more and more people were convinced. We may look out of the window and still find it hard to believe that the world is really round but even the most sceptical of us believe the evidence of the astronaut's camera. We respect that the photographs taken from his different viewpoint provide as much proof as we need to believe that the world is round.

The degree to which one believes in a theory depends on one's own knowledge, frame of reference and culture. The culture gap between doctors and ordinary people is vast. Doctors have had years and years of indoctrination into the supremacy of science over common sense, and into the superiority of hospital birth over home birth. We should not be too hard on them.

There are both historical and current examples of scientific narrow mindedness.

Puerperal fever
The classic example of flat earth thinking in obstetrics is the cause of puerperal fever. As early as 1843 an American doctor, Oliver Wendell Holmes, who happened also to be a poet (further proof of the need for sensitivity in science)

published a paper entitled: "On the Contagiousness of Puerperal Fever". Four years later Dr Ignaz Semmelweis wrote that "Puerperal Fever is caused by conveyance to the pregnant woman of putrid particles derived from living organisms, through the agency of the examining fingers". In other words, puerperal fever was a disease caused by medicine itself, an infection carried from woman to woman on the hands of surgeons and midwives. Mortality rates from puerperal fever varied from hospital to hospital and from doctor to doctor. In the days before antibiotics prevention was the only option available. Semmelweis advised doctors to wash their hands in chloride of lime between each delivery. The doctors considered this advice impertinent, categorically refusing to believe themselves capable of bringing death to their patients. Death rates did not start to fall until the end of the century. Puerperal fever remained a risk until the 1930s. Even today women die of septic abortions – and not only from back street abortionists.

Blind babies

In the early 1940s a new disease appeared out of the blue. Apparently healthy babies a few months old suddenly became blind. An epidemic started in America and by 1945 one doctor had identified 117 cases. Then the epidemic spread to Britain, it escalated with the advent of the NHS. This turned out to be another disease caused by hospital treatment. The doctors were mystified and eventually discovered what was happening to the babies' eyes and labelled the disease retrolental fibroplasia. The label did not help with finding out why babies were going blind. Nor did it explain why only premature babies suffered. Again the incidence varied from hospital to hospital and even from ward to ward. But the answer when it came was simple. The babies were being blinded by overzealous care. In high-tech hospitals premature babies were nursed in incubators and given extra supplies of oxygen to prevent oxygen starvation. And you can't have too much of a good thing. You can! The extra oxygen caused abnormal eye development and some of the babies became blind. Ten thousand of them. The link with oxygen was first mooted in 1951 and by 1955 the epidemic was abating as oxygen therapy was delivered less intensively and over shorter periods. But it took time to change hospital practice, night nurses would surreptitiously increase oxygen, just as they surreptitiously feed babies today while their mothers are asleep.

But doctors found that whereas too much oxygen risked blinding their charges, too little – and the babies suffered oxygen starvation. One doctor estimated that for every baby who was spared oxygen therapy and thus retained his sight, 16 died from respiratory distress and oxygen starvation. These risks must still be balanced, even today. Man cannot design the perfect incubator, it already exists, it is called woman. We need to reduce the risk of prematurity itself rather than attempt to make better incubators. We must relieve pregnant women from unnecessary stress.

Cot Death – The Facts

Multifactorial theory

The greatest fear of any new mother is that she will find her baby dead in his cot, for no apparent reason. The sudden infant death syndrome (SIDS) is largely preventable. It belongs in this particular book because it has been linked, among other factors, with premature delivery, caesarean section and inadequate maternal behaviour. In the developing world it is virtually unheard of but in the developed world it is associated with birth order in the family, spacing between births, social class, poverty and even the weather. The government and one cot death charity have made much of the link with sleeping position. Cot deaths have fallen by a half since mothers were advised to put their babies to sleep on their backs. However, sleeping position is just another factor in cot death which is still said to have multifactorial causes. We can call this classic collection of epidemiological evidence the multifactorial theory. But the multifactorial theory has now been superseded by a single theory that unites nearly all the other evidence.

Toxic gas theory

In 1989 Barry Richardson, an industrial chemist discovered, quite by chance, that cot mattresses were treated with certain industrial chemicals, flame retardants and plasticisers, which contained chemical compounds of phosphorus and antimony and even traces of arsenic. Some common household fungi, like those on mouldy cheese, can digest these compounds and breathe out phosphine, stibine and arsine gases as waste products, just as we breathe out carbon dioxide. Phosphine, stibine and arsine gases are toxic gases which interfere with heart and lung function. They are heavier than air and tend to gravitate downwards to lie at the surface of the mattress or fill the holes in aerated mattresses. Household fungi need warmth, moisture and a food supply to survive and multiply. Babies supply the warmth and the moisture, and the cot mattress itself supplies the food in the form of the very material of the mattress itself. Over time, as the cot mattress is warmed up by the baby, the fungi become more prolific and spread and eventually enough gases may be generated to kill the baby, particularly if he sleeps on his front with his mouth and nose close to the gases. More and more fungi convert more and more of the potentially poisonous compounds into poisonous gases.

Mr Richardson arranged for the blood of babies who had died a cot death to be assayed, and assays showed higher than normal traces of the poison antimony; he tested samples of mattresses on which babies had died and found signs of fungal infestation, particularly in the area affected by the warmth and perspiration of the baby. He found visual evidence of plasticiser deterioration – the mattresses had become more brittle where the baby had been. My own second-hand carry cot showed a typical pattern of plasticiser deterioration. There was a hard brittle patch in the middle of the inside of the front panel, surrounded by rays of softer plastic. We were lucky that our firstborn grew out of the carry cot quickly enough to avoid a cot death, and that there was a three and a half year gap before the next baby came. But others are not so lucky. Cot death is now the single most common cause of infant death and nearly all cot deaths are preventable.

Toxic gases damage nerves, particularly the vagus nerve which innervates the lungs and heart. Cot death babies simply stop breathing. Our bodies are able to deal with a certain amount of poison but there comes a point when they are overwhelmed by poisons and death ensues. This point will be reached earlier in babies with congenital weaknesses. Premature babies and babies born by caesarean section are likely to have poorer lung function owing to inadequate supplies of cortisol at birth and will therefore be more likely to succumb to cot death.

Unknown to the cot death researchers, the common name for the syndrome already hinted at the cause of death.

The cover-up

According to my reasoning the evidence presented above should be enough in itself to warn parents of the possible risks of cot mattresses. Any contaminated mattress could be in effect a time bomb. The solution is simple, parents should buy a new mattress for each new baby or else totally enclose a second-hand mattress in polythene. But, according to one major cot death charity, and according to the government, the theory was not proven beyond reasonable doubt. It was too soon to warn parents that their babies might die on an old mattress. As lately as 1992 the said charity and the government, for reasons known only to themselves, did not want parents to find out about the toxic gas theory of cot death. Even if it were proved conclusively that mattresses did *not* cause cot death, which I believe is impossible given the lack of any other plausible theory and the strength of the evidence outlined above, what harm would have been done? This seems to be flat earth thinking at its very worst.

The charity and the government both knew of the existence of the theory well before distributing leaflets on how to prevent cot deaths in the autumn of 1991: "Back to Sleep" from the Department of Health, and "Reducing the Risks of Cot Death" from the charity. Neither leaflet so much as hinted at the possible role of the cot mattress in causing cot death. Government laboratories attempted to replicate the toxic gas findings and found enough evidence of fungoid activity to justify further research. The charity set up an independent team and failed to replicate Mr Richardson's results which, according to them: "had not been carried out under laboratory conditions"! Neither considered that there was enough evidence even to *warn* parents that cot mattresses *might* be involved in cot death. How much evidence is necessary before scientific findings can be aired in public? When will parents be treated as responsible adults, given the facts, and allowed to decide important issues for themselves?

Ethnic differences and sleeping position

Cot death is virtually unique to the Western world which sleeps babies in cots. Other babies at risk are those who sleep on sheep skins. New Zealand has a particularly high rate of cot death but regional variations correlate highly with natural arsenic levels in sheep grazing areas, arsenic is ingested with grass and gets into the fleece. Researchers in New Zealand were the first to find the link between sleeping position and cot death. However, sleeping position is a secondary factor.

Many ethnic groups strongly reject advice to sleep their babies on their backs because of the increased risk of choking. Moreover, the so-called uncivilised mothers are far less likely to use cots at all – they carry their babies around swaddled close to them by day and sleep in the same place at night. The cot death charity is pursuing the idea that ethnic minorities are less at risk because infants have more physical stimulation. This is a likely secondary factor; stimulation strengthens the immune system and may well raise the threshold of adverse reactions to all manner of environmental invasions – including toxic gases. Michel Odent explores this enormous new research area in his book *Primal Health*.

Evidence
Since the chemical evidence seems to be considered controversial by the government and the charity, I will consider only the evidence agreed by both sides: the statistical probabilities of the various factors involved. But I will start from an opposing viewpoint, namely that second-hand mattresses, quite possibly, could be contaminated by fungi that may have the ability to metabolise chemical compounds containing the elements phosphorus and antimony, compounds which we know are put into the plastic coverings of mattresses as flame retardants and plasticisers. We can now make predictions about the babies who would be most at risk of cot death. The theory predicts that fungal infestation will be highest and most active on recently used mattresses.

1. We would expect to find deaths highest in societies that put their babies to sleep on Western style mattresses.

They are. Cot death is virtually unknown among Bangladeshi families in Cardiff but the rate for white babies reflects the rate for the UK as a whole. The Bangladeshi mothers do not use Western style cot mattresses. At night babies tend to sleep with their parents, and during the day they are laid down to sleep in any convenient place on improvised bedding, just as Western mothers make do when they are away from home with no available cot.

2. We would expect to find more deaths among second, third and fourth babies in the same family.

There are. The statistical risk of cot death increases with family size, and the closer the temporal spacing between children, the higher the risk. The risk for the third baby of a teenage mother, a mother who must have had her children very close together, is *eight times* as high as the average risk.

3. We would expect to find more deaths in poorer families who relied on the second-hand market for their baby equipment.

There are. Babies of impoverished, young and single mothers are most at risk.

4. *We would expect to find that babies who sleep on their tummy are more likely to die than babies sleeping on their back.*

Everyone agrees that this is the case. The cot death rate has halved since the "Back to Sleep" campaign was launched.

The total infant mortality rate could be half the 1989 rate if only the charity and the government could tell mothers that old mattresses can kill babies. At the time of writing (November 1992) the charity is still implying that putting babies to sleep on their back is the best way to prevent cot death.

Like the toxic gas theory, my stress and childbirth theory has yet to be proved beyond all doubt, and like the toxic gas theory, given enough publicity, and the will to change, it could have a startling effect on the infant mortality rate.

13   Hope For The Future

May the obstetricians forget about the powers, passage, passenger, parturition and puerperium and let them put the people back into childbirth.

I hope that all who have read thus far will share my belief that the modern approach to childbirth is fundamentally wrong and recognise that change is imperative if we are to improve the lot of labouring women, their children and their families in the future. There is a long road to travel. We must retrace our steps right back to the Garden of Eden to remove the very real fears that men and women have of childbirth, and travel forward again to meet the needs of our modern world and our natural demand for safe, painfree childbirth and the best possible start to life for our children.

The psychology of pregnancy, labour and bonding is in its infancy and is ignored by obstetricians who continue to see birth in engineering terms, its success measured only by perinatal mortality and morbidity rates. The intuitive skills of midwives tend to be disparaged and the mother's feelings trampled underfoot. Communications skills have only recently entered the medical students' curriculum and still tend to be regarded as a waste of time for those not intending to become GPs or psychiatrists. Hospitals are busy places and obstetricians can be impatient, often preferring to intervene in normal labour before midwives or mothers think it necessary. Human nature and medical politics being what they are, the obstetricians' interests are all too often focused on power, status and money rather than the needs of their patients. It was a grave mistake historically to link together obstetrics and gynaecology as medical specialties and an even graver mistake to concentrate childbirth in large teaching hospitals, where there is a never ending supply of students to be given experience in techniques of intervention and surgery.

Gynaecology is concerned with sick women whereas obstetrics concerns predominantly healthy women. A doctor who deals with both sick and healthy women in the course of the working day in the hospital environment will tend to regard all his patients as sick. The midwives' view of birth is far more positive since they deal only with healthy women, being forced to hand over responsibility to their medical colleagues at the first hint of trouble, and the reasons for transferring responsibility become ever more trivial as the boundary between normal and abnormal childbirth is redefined to include more and more women.

Women have paid for civilisation with their very bodies. The price is pain, loss of personal fulfilment in childbirth, and a higher risk of mortality and disease. The physical outcome may be better now for mother and child, although gross interference with the natural hormones of labour has largely unrecognised consequences, but the psychological outcome is appalling and has a direct bearing on society as a whole.

Violence breeds violence. By subjecting our children to violence at birth are we condemning them to a life of violence? Are we giving them a false picture of the world as an unfriendly, clinical, noisy place where technology reigns supreme and human relationships take the back seat?

How do we start to reform childbirth and lying-in? How do we, the mothers, educate the educators when the system is so geared towards the medical model? Many groups have been set up for this purpose but some of these have been so convinced by the obstetricians' arguments that they have changed sides and now spend their resources fighting for more neonatal cots, more foetal monitors and epidurals on demand. The outlets for medical propaganda are many, but mothers are still denied a platform for their views. Despite the support of mothers and midwives, the Winterton Report has done nothing to alter the status quo. All the signs are that the present hospital system will shamble its way along for the foreseeable future. Home birth supporters are still regarded as cranks risking their babies' lives for the so-called dubious psychological benefits of natural birth.

When will the establishment stop seeing women as pawns on the production lines of vast maternity hospitals and start to consider their real needs? Curtains and wallpaper in labour rooms, a quick cuddle after the birth and a more relaxed attitude to rooming-in seem to be the sum total of achievements in the last decade – clear proof that women are being ignored.

Block booking at antenatal clinics, the chief complaint of all pregnant women, is still the norm. Is the doctor's time so very precious that he has to have a string of women waiting to see him just in case one does not turn up? If the large hospitals cannot even manage to organise antenatal clinics better are they fit to be taking control of childbirth at all? What is being done to respond to fathers' needs? Has anyone even asked fathers what they want for their families? Perhaps a fathers' pressure group would have more influence over the male-dominated hospital system.

The inequalities between men and women are set right from the beginning of life when males control childbirth instead of women. Medical childbirth is a self-perpetuating system of male dominance over women.

Medical institutions such as the Royal College of Obstetricians and Gynaecologists have always put their members' interests first and have a strong platform from which to proclaim their views. Doctors being male professionals have a high social status; their professional opinions are taken as gospel and respected by the predominantly male establishment; in virtually any enquiry into matters pertaining to health, they have the louder voice, regardless of the fact that in everyday life childcare is women's business; they are regarded as scientists and their pontifications are thus seen to be grounded in fact – whether or not the facts bear out their opinions; they can bend ears in high places to achieve their ends. How are midwives and mothers, the labourers themselves, to counteract this barrage of professional interest? Women form pressure groups but usually fail to make any major impact on society unless they can attract a big name or take advantage of a current news story.

Individual mothers can, however, take strike action, they can vote with their feet and refuse to go to hospital at all.

My feeling is that we must get the GPs on our side. The GP is nearly always the first point of contact with the maternity services. If we could only persuade GPs to ask "And would you like to have this baby at home or in hospital?" instead of "Which hospital do you want to go to?" the battle would be nearly over.

GPs have lost nearly as much as midwives in the trend towards hospital delivery and have a lot to gain from reclaiming home birth for their patients. Earlier this century they may have received their preliminary training in medical schools but they learnt how to be a GP on the job. Most of their obstetric experience came from attending home births. Today GPs only ever learn high-tech obstetrics, with the emphasis being on complicated labours – normal births are left to the midwives. All the students are rushed in to observe an interesting face presentation; none are rushed in to observe a natural birth. Too few women have home births which would provide training opportunities for GPs or for midwives. Training is grossly distorted towards the high-tech model.

GPs are denied one of the most joyful parts of general practice, that of welcoming their new patients into the world. Birth was traditionally the time when the family doctor became a family friend, a person whose advice could be trusted. How many people can see their GP as a family friend today? No amount of communication skills and education can replace friendship resulting from the profound shared experience of a major event such as birth or death, and few GPs and young adults share such an experience; it is more likely to come later in life with the illnesses of old age. If GPs and women learnt to trust each other better and to talk to each other openly, perhaps there would be fewer unnecessary GP prescriptions for tranquillizers, cold cures and antibiotics and less referrals to hospital for needless investigations or psychiatric problems. We must enlist the GPs in our struggle for a devolution of power from the hospital-based system.

Education for all

Education to remove everyone's fear that something may go wrong is the very first step to take and removing other causes of stress in childbirth would then follow close behind. I have written this book primarily for mothers since they have the most to gain from learning how their own bodies work in labour. Women need to know the facts before they can give informed consent to intervention in childbirth; they need to know the facts so that they can take an active role in deciding how and where to labour. They need to know the fact that it is wiser and safer not to hand over control of their bodies to other people.

Professionals need even more education to counteract the misinformation that has passed for science in recent years. They need to learn how to trust women's instincts in labour and facilitate the process rather than take over completely. They need to become less professional and more human in their attitude, they need to learn respect for the women they serve. They need to learn how to teach women the physical importance of active *self-management* of labour and how to encourage rather than discourage women to take control of labour into their own hands.

Immediate action

Education apart, what can we do now to turn the tide? An obvious solution is to encourage GP unit and home birth – but who is to supervise it? Fortunately, even today there are still a few brave independent midwives prepared to risk their livelihood and all their worldly goods (through litigation) in order to enable women to give birth at home; there are still a few enlightened GPs willing to take on home births.

In England we are very fortunate that the right to choose where to labour is inscribed on the statute book. Every woman wanting a home birth is legally entitled to one and the NHS is compelled to provide a midwife. There is no legal requirement for the presence of a doctor although a midwife is required to call for medical assistance when she deems it necessary, and any doctor called by a midwife has a legal duty to attend.

If your baby is due tomorrow and you decide to have a home birth instead of a hospital birth you can go to your GP and ask him to instruct the Health Authority to send a midwife. He may very well refuse to cover your labour himself, that is his right; he may well pull out all the stops to try to dissuade you, but you can have your baby at home – that is your right, enshrined in law. Changing your mind at the eleventh hour is a perfectly sensible decision to take. If you would feel happier at home, have the baby at home.

If you still feel wary about home birth, at least shun large teaching hospitals like the plague and go to a GP unit. Get to know all the midwives there during your pregnancy and trust them to help you to deliver your baby. At all costs avoid interference; practice saying "no" to yourself three times before breakfast. Then, when you need to, you can say "no". Carry on saying it until someone hears and listens. The baby is in your body, you are his mother and he is your responsibility. You will be doing the work, the professionals are there to help you to do it better, not to do it for you.

You can always threaten to sue for physical assault if your wishes are not adhered to. Threatening litigation is very much the last resort but it does work; it allowed me to go home with our daughter the day after a normal delivery, despite a posse of professionals crowded into a small room trying to convince me of the dangers of going home. The only concrete example of a danger was that I was Rhesus negative and my daughter Rhesus positive – all that was required was a simple injection. I could not go home because they were treating me so nicely – I had been given an amenity bed. Only three years later they were sending all mothers home as soon as possible owing to shortage of beds. Policy is determined by the number of available beds rather than by need.

Fear of Litigation

Confrontational obstetrics is not, however, the best way forward to achieve my dream of joyful childbirth for all. GPs often refuse to cover home birth for fear of litigation should something go wrong; midwives call in the doctors too readily and follow the rule book too closely for fear of losing their livelihood should something go wrong; obstetricians intervene too readily in normal labour for fear of litigation should something go wrong. Fear of litigation should something go wrong has itself become the underlying cause of the barbarism of civilised childbirth. We are already following the Americans down the path of litigation; there is a shortage of obstetricians because the insurance premiums are too high. (Personally I feel that this shortage will work to our ultimate advantage, but that will a long time in the future.) Compensation orders of hundreds of thousands of pounds are made whenever the lawyers can prove that an obstetrician failed to do something that he could have done.

We have been looking down the wrong end of a telescope. If the obstetricians had their wits about them they could so easily prove that birth accidents occur more often through over-zealous intervention than through neglect. Moreover, accidents of birth caused by genetic defects have no monetary compensation in our society. Why should the victim of birth trauma fare so much better financially than the victim of a genetic accident of birth? Who is to say whether a condition is congenital, genetic or medically-induced? It has been said many times before that the chief beneficiaries of litigation are the lawyers. The NHS needs all the money it can get to care for an ageing population; why waste money on lining the pockets of lawyers? The only sensible solution for obstetrics, where intervention is contraindicated in virtually every situation, is no-fault compensation.

No-fault compensation

No-fault compensation would probably halve the perinatal mortality rate at a stroke and save countless children from disability caused by unnecessary intervention. It could save up to a fifth of mothers from major abdominal surgery, it could save countless more from postnatal depression and increase the quality of family life for years to come, eventually heralding a less violent society. It would save the NHS millions of pounds in lawyers fees, compensation orders, maternity beds and special-care cots. No-fault compensation would go a long way towards eliminating stress in childbirth and is the only rational way forward. The case for the association between intervention and perinatal mortality has already been proved statistically and this book gives the scientific foundations for the observed facts. No-fault compensation could revolutionise childbirth. The thin end of the wedge argument used against no-fault compensation in this country – that it would lead to no-fault compensation in other areas of medicine – could easily be countered by stating the simple fact that childbirth is a normal, natural event, not a medical emergency.

Hospital childbirth

Hospital childbirth is here to stay for the foreseeable future, but how much better it could be. A change of attitude to users is the first requirement. The chief advantage private hospitals have over NHS hospitals is in the attitude of staff towards patients. Patients are respected in the private sector, if only because their money pays the bills. There may be little to choose from regarding physical quality of care but the private patient is at least encouraged to retain his self-respect, which is the first thing to be lost when walking through the doors of a large maternity hospital. It is far harder to bully people who pay for their treatment directly rather than through the taxation system.

How can we effect a shift of attitudes? There are three main ways. First by widening choice and thus competition between hospitals, second by having more but smaller maternity units and third by encouraging personal relationships to develop between staff and the women they care for – introducing a named midwife approach to maternity services.

Consumer-led services

NHS Trust hospitals already have to sell their services to GPs and maternity hospitals should sell their services directly to mothers. If mothers were carrying a maternity voucher for whatever it costs to have a baby in the NHS in their pocket on their first antenatal visit, the tables would be turned. Hospitals would then start to respect mothers more and compete with each other at giving mothers what they need above all else – freedom from stress and freedom of movement – control over their own labour.

It could be said with some justification that a consumer-oriented system does not appear to work in America, but in America the obstetricians' lobby is even more powerful. US obstetricians have car stickers proclaiming that home delivery is for pizzas. In the USA choice is to a large extent determined by the services health insurance companies are willing to cover. Low-tech birthing centres have been set up and are safe and popular among the women who use them but some health insurance companies refuse to pay for treatment. Jessica Mitford has done a great service for American women in exposing the shortcomings of their maternity services. Certainly the British system could be a lot worse – but it could be infinitely better.

Continuity of care in hospital services

Continuity of care is impossible while antenatal care is organised around the obstetrician who is overseeing vastly more women than he can expect to care for in labour. A significant step towards providing real continuity of care would be to break down the staffing barriers between the labour ward and antenatal clinics and organise antenatal clinics around pairs of midwives who would be responsible for individual women throughout antenatal care and during labour itself. Instead of being booked into a consultant's antenatal clinic and seeing him at the end of the production line, a woman would see one of the two midwives who will actually deliver her baby. This would enable mothers and midwives alike to build a sound relationship and learn to trust each other well before labour. Thus a woman entering hospital in labour would be cared for by someone she knew well and could work with, who respected her wishes and had already discussed options for labour.

Misunderstandings would be far less common. The midwife delivering the baby need not rely so heavily on notes made by other people and failures in communication, so often the cause of human problems, could be virtually eliminated. Clashes of personality could be dealt with simply by a woman moving to a different team. As well as being of infinite benefit to labouring women, job satisfaction would be significantly enhanced for midwives and perhaps fewer would leave the profession so soon after training (two thirds of trained midwives do not practice). This is perhaps unthinkable for a society convinced that the only people fit to be responsible for childbirth are consultant obstetricians. Women still probably feel that they should see the consultant at each visit.

Perhaps for the moment the midwives could still work under a consultant, and women could then decide whether or not they wanted to see the consultant himself on antenatal visits, with midwives referring only those who needed a medical opinion for some specific problem. Such a scheme has already been outlined in *The Named Midwife*, a report from the Patient's Charter Group. It requires no new facilities but would probably involve paying midwives more for extra responsibility. There is little doubt, however, that the extra costs would be recouped in savings made in consultants' time, in unnecessary interventions and prevention of problems in labour and after. Caroline Flint has outined the practicalities of such a scheme, but her name cannot even be mentioned in one maternity hospital without howls of protest from midwives themselves!

The barriers between hospital and community staff would be broken down if the named midwife also provided postnatal care, and eventually responsibility for birth itself would be transferred to the community. Community midwives are already involved in some antenatal care, some home births, the domino system, and postnatal care. We need a half-way house towards home birth: local birth centres with a few maternity beds staffed by midwives to which all but the very highest risk women would go for antenatal care thus getting to know all the staff and already feeling at home when the time comes for labour. During labour itself there could be an obstetrician on call and willing to perform forceps deliveries on site rather than assuming the worst and transferring mothers to consultant units. Keeping lower risk women out of consultant units would have the added advantage of reducing them in size so that a high-risk woman would feel less like a product on a conveyor belt. Familiarity with both the staff and the place would be an enormous improvement in childbirth for all women, wheresoever that place may be.

At the moment hospital care is seen as superior to community care, probably as a result of the twentieth century conviction that the more money spent on a system, and the more sophisticated technology there is, the better it must be. In order to humanise services a fundamental change of attitude is required, an attitude which puts personal relationships above money and technology.

Preventing prematurity

A more personal approach to antenatal care would probably reap large financial rewards in preventing prematurity. Women who have poor emotional support during pregnancy are more likely to give birth prematurely, and care by named midwives would automatically give pregnant women support by fostering closer interpersonal links. There needs to be much more psychological input into midwives' training so that they are better able to recognise warning signs of impending problems, social and psychological as well as physical. If a midwife were to become a personal friend then women would find her more approachable and feel more able to ask her advice about things she thought too trivial to bother hospital staff, and problems would then be recognised before they became out of hand. Such a midwife would also be better equipped to care emotionally for a woman who miscarried, bore a damaged baby or suffered a stillbirth. This is perhaps asking a lot of any human being. The emotional strains on the midwife herself would be higher but these would be offset by the emotional rewards.

Is there still a place for obstetricians and technology?

We need not throw out the baby with the bath water. Despite my generally negative attitude to it, technology has a place – but it should be kept in its place, as a servant and not a master. Similarly obstetricians could become servants instead of masters of labouring women. Caesarean sections are necessary for transverse lie and placenta praevia, but the timing of the operation could still be decided by the baby; it is madness to decide the date weeks in advance. Medical research should be directed at finding ways of reducing the caesarean section rate which could probably come down to as little as 1%. Let us develop an obstetric flying squad appropriate for home births to remove residual fears that something more could have been done in hospital. Let medical technology invent a portable incubator to transfer sick babies to hospital if necessary. Bring back the Pinard stethoscope and birthing stool and throw away the foetal monitor. Is this really such a pipe dream? Am I crying for the moon? If such measures are technically possible then the last remaining source of stress in childbirth would be removed and the final fear conquered.

Who should manage childbirth?

Childbirth is a natural physiological process. No one, man or woman, would dream of telling a woman how to menstruate – the very idea is absurd and yet everyday hundreds of women up and down the country are being told how to labour by men. No man but the father has any place in childbirth itself; even the role of the GP in normal labour becomes questionable. When the first male midwife qualified there was a general feeling of unease that a man should become intimately concerned with women in labour but few have questioned the right of male doctors to manage labour. Childbirth is women's labour, and who but a woman can possibly understand the rhythmical workings of her body? I would like to see the Royal College of Obstetricians and Gynaecologists gradually becoming an all female body, with entry requirements to include

208

personal experience of childbirth. We would end up with a service provided by mothers for mothers.

Let us put the mother back into childbirth. Let us have tears of joy instead of tears of sorrow. Let us give birth joyfully and happily at home.

General Sources

Barrington E J W (1964). *Hormones and Evolution*, Unibooks.

Brook D (1976). *Naturebirth*, Heinemann, Penguin.

Broster L R (1945). *Endocrine Man*, Heinemann.

Clark-Kennedy A E (1969). *Man, Medicine and Morality*, Faber and Faber.

Coon C S (1957). *The History of Man*, Jonathan Cape.

Dawkins R (1986). *The Blind Watchmaker*, Longman.

Dawkins R (1982). *The Extended Phenotype*, Oxford.

Harrison R J (1969). *Reproduction and Man*, Oliver and Boyd.

Hutt C (1972). *Males and Females*, Penguin.

Johnson M and Everitt B (1984). *Essential Reproduction*, Blackwell.

Myle's Textbook for Midwives, (1989). 11th edn, eds V R Bennett and L K Brown.

Savage W (1986). *A Savage Enquiry*, Virago.

Spielberger C (1979). *Understanding Stress and Anxiety*, Harper and Row.

Wesson N (1990). *Home Birth, a practical guide*, Optima.

References

Asher, R (1972). *Talking Sense*, Pitman Medical.

Backon J (1989). *Medical Hypotheses*, **28**, 213-214.

Bourne G (1989). *Pregnancy*, Pan.

British National Formulary, March 1989.

Browning *et al* (1983). *British Journal of Obstetrics and Gynaecology*, **90**, 1147-51.

Burns J K (1992). *Journal of Psychosomatic Obstetrics and Gynaecology*, **11**, 37-49.

Campbell R and MacFarlane A (1987). *Where to be born? The debate and the evidence*, National Perinatal Epidemiology Unit, Radcliffe Infirmary, Oxford.

Carlson N R (1991). *The Physiology of Behaviour*, Allyn and Bacon.

Coleman V (1988). *The Health Scandal*, Sidgwick and Jackson.

Conley A J and Mason J I (1990). In *Endocrinology of Pregnancy*, ed S Franks, Ballière Tindall.

Cooper W (1976). *No Change*, Arrow.

Csapo A (1961). in *Progesterone and the Defence Mechanism of Pregnancy*, eds G E W Wolstenholme and M P Cameron, Churchill.

Dally A (1991). *Women under the Knife*, Hutchinson Radius.

Dalton K (1984). *The Premenstrual Syndrome and Progesterone Therapy*. William Heinemann Medical Books.

Dawkins R (1976). *The Selfish Gene*, 2nd edn, Oxford University Press.

Devorshak-Harvey E (1988). *Neuroendocrinology*, **48**, 584-90.

Dick-Read G (1942). *Childbirth Without Fear*, Heinemann.

Elstein M and Chantler E N (1990). in *The Scientific Foundations of Obstetrics and Gynaecology*, Butterworth/Heinemann.

Facchinetti F *et al* (1982). *Gynecologic and Obstetric Investigation*, **13**, 155-163.

Flint C (1992). *Name, set and match*, paper given at the Forum on Maternity and the Newborn.

Figuero J P *et al* (1989). *American Journal of Obstetrics and Gynecology*, **161**, 481-6.

Garai J, Vertes M and Kovacs S (1989). *Journal of Steroid Biochemistry*, **32**, 433-438.

Goland *et al* (1988). *American Journal of Obstetrics and Gynecology*, **159**, 884-890.

Goldberg J (1989). *Anatomy of a Scientific Discovery*, Bantam Books.

HMSO (1992). House of Commons Health Committee report.

Hoffman D L *et al* (1984). *American Journal of Obstetrics and Gynecology*, **150**, 492-6.

Homer *et al* (1990). *American Journal of Public Health*, **80**, 173-7.

Honnebier M B *et al* (1989). *Endocrinology*, **125**, 1498-1503.

Huntingford P (1984). *Birth Right, The parents' choice*, BBC.

Kauppila A, Tuimala R and Haapalauti J (1974). *Journal of Obstetrics and Gynaecology of the British Commonwealth*, **81**, 691-694.

Kitzinger J (1989). in *Politics of Maternity Care*, Clarendon.

Kitzinger S (1979). *Birth at Home*. Oxford.

Kosterlitz A H and Hughes J (1975). *Nature*, **258**, 577.

Laatikainen T J (1991). *Annals of Medicine*, **23**, 489-96.

Läpple, M (1988). *Zentralblatt Fur Gynakologie*, **110**, 325-35.

Leng G *et al* (1988). *Journal of Reproduction and Fertility*, **84**, 345-56.

Levenson R W (1988).in *Social Psychophsiology and Emotion*, ed H L Wagner, John Wiley and Sons.

Llewellyn-Jones, D (1990). *Fundamentals of Obstetrics and Gynaecology, Part I Obstetrics*, Faber and Faber.

Low K G *et al (1989)*. *Molecular Endocrinology*, **3**, 852-7.

Margioris *et al* (1988). *Journal of Clinical Endocrinology and Metabolism*, **66**, 922-26.

McLaren (1961). in *Progesterone and the Defence Mechanism of Pregnancy*, eds G E W Wolstenholme and M P Cameron, Churchill.

Mendelson C R and Boggaram V (1990). in *Endocrinology of Pregnancy*, ed S Franks, Ballière Tindall.

Mitford J (1992). *The American Way of Birth*, Gollanz.

Morgan E (1972). *The Descent of Woman*, Souvenir Press.

Morgan B M *et al* (1984). *British Journal of Obstetrics and Gynaecology*, **91**, 624-628.

Murphy B (1979). in *Interaction within the Brain-Pituitary-Adrenocortical System*, eds M J Jones, B Gillham, M F Dallman and S Chattopadhyay, Academic Press.

Nathan P (1990). in *The Oxford Companion to the Mind*, ed R L Gregory, Oxford University Press, p 516.

O'Brien M (1978). *Journal of the Royal College of General Practitioners*, **28**, 460-466.

Odent M (1986). *Primal Health*, Century Hutchinson.

O'Driscoll K and Meagher D (1986). *The Active Management of Labour*, 2nd edn, Ballière Tindall.

Ohia S E and Laniyonu (1989). *Journal of Pharmacy and Pharmacology*, **41**, 168-172.

Olster DH and Blaustein JD (1990). *Journal of Neurobiology*, **21**, 768-80.

Omer H and Everly G S (1988). *American Journal of Psychiatry*, **145**, 1507-13.

Parsons B (1975). *Expectant Fathers*, Robert Yeatman Ltd.

Pearsall R (1969). *The Worm in the Bud*, Pelican edn (1971).

Philipp, E (1988). *Caesareans*, Sidgwick and Jackson.

Pickles V R and Fitzpatrick R J (1966). *Endogenous Substances affecting the Myometrium*. Cambridge University Press.

Plotnikoff N P and Murgo A J (1985). *Federation Proceedings*, **44**, 91.

Racey P A (1981). in *Environmental Factors in Mammalian Reproduction*, eds B Gilmore and B Cook, Macmillan.

Romero R et al (1988). *American Journal of Obstetrics and Gynecology*, **159**, 657-60.

Rose K J (1988). *The Body in Time*, Wiley Science Editions, p 100.

Russell J A et al (1989). *Journal of Endocrinology*, **121**, 521-36.

Shaarawy et al, (1991). *Fertility and Sterility*, **56**, 248-53.

Scheinin M et al (1990). *Acta Anaesthesiologica Scandinavica*, **43**, 640-4.

Suda et al (1978). *Science*, **202**, 221-3.

Taneike et al (1991). *Biology of Reproduction*, **45**, 831-40.

Tew, Marjorie (1990) *Safer Childbirth?* Chapman and Hall.

Trowell, J (1982). cited in *Politics of Maternity Care*, ed J Garcia, R Kilpatrick and M Richards, Clarendon Paperbacks.

Verney T and Kelly J (1981). *The Secret Life of the Unborn Child*, Summit Books, USA; English edn Sphere (1982).

Vertes M, Pamer Z and Garai J (1986). *Journal of Steroid Biochemistry*, **24**, 235-8).

Women's Co-operative Guild (1915). *Maternity: Letters from Working Women*, ed M Llewelyn Davies; new edn (1978) ed G Dallas, Virago.

Glossary

Hormones

Act hormone, the *make cortisol* message.

androgens, predominantly male sex hormones including testosterone. Produced in the adrenal gland and testicles.

adrenaline sudden stress hormone produced in the adrenal gland as a response to a nervous signal from the brain. Acts in the body as a biochemical bridge between nerve cells.

adrenocorticotropic hormone, ACT hormone, the *release cortisol* message, one of the POMC hormones, secreted by the pituitary gland.

ß-endorphin, a natural opium-like hormone, see page 61.

cortisol, arousal hormone produced in the adrenal gland as a response to ACT hormone from the pituitary.

CRF, corticotropin releasing hormone, the *release ACT hormone* message, also releases the other POMC hormones.

growth hormone, secreted to promote normal growth, stopped by ß-endorphin. Can be given by doctors to speed up growth in small children.

luteinising hormone, (LH), the *make oestrogen* message, secreted by the pituitary gland on a hormonal instruction from the hypothalamus (GnRH, gonadotropin releasing hormone).

met-enkephalin, a small section of the ß-endorphin molecule with similar effects but short-lived. Released in conjunction with oxytocin from the pituitary gland.

MSH, melanocyte stimulating hormone, One of the POMC hormones.

noradrenaline, sudden stress hormone, also a neurotransmitter in the brain.

oestrogens, female steroid sex hormones found throughout the animal kingdom. Oestrogens exist in various forms, some forms have stronger effects than others. Produced mainly in the ovaries but also sometimes in the placenta and the adrenal glands.

oxytocin, pituitary hormone released as a response to stretching the cervix, vagina and nipples.

prolactin, the nest-building, grooming and milk-making hormone. Switched on by ß-endorphin and oxytocin.

pro-opiomelanocortin, POMC, a bundle of hormones split apart to produce, among other substances, ACT hormone, MSH and beta-endorphin. Released by CRF and progesterone. See page 62.

progesterone, the pregnancy hormone. Produced by the ruptured egg follicle in the ovary and the placenta. A precursor to other steroid hormones in the adrenal gland. See pages 74 and 79.

prostaglandins, local hormones manufactured and used locally, involved in many aspects of reproduction including intercourse, menstruation and labour. Also involved in the body's immune reaction to foreign bodies. The various types of prostaglandins differ in their ability to elicit uterine contractions.

relaxin, a hormone secreted at menstruation and during pregnancy, loosens joints making the birth canal more pliable.

steroid hormones, small simple hormones found throughout the animal kingdom, one steroid hormone can be changed to another by enzymes that add or take away atoms of hydrogen or oxygen. Manufactured from cholesterol in the adrenal glands, testicles, ovaries and placenta. In theory any steroid hormone-producing gland can manufacture all the steroid hormones. In practice hormones made depend on enzymes available at the relevant gland. See page 74.

testosterone, the aggression hormone, a male sex hormone produced in the testicles in men and in the adrenal gland in women.

General

amino acid, constituent molecules of proteins. There are about 22 different amino acids in living cells, different combinations of amino acids make different proteins.

amniotic fluid, the waters, the fluid surrounding the baby *in utero*, contained in two layers of membranes, the chorion and the amnion. As well as protecting the foetus, the fluid and the membranes manufacture hormones.

anaesthesia, numbness.

analgesia, pain relief.

antepartum, before birth.

anthropology, the study of man.

ARM, artificial rupture of the membranes surrounding the baby *in utero*.

autonomic nervous system, that part of the nervous system controlling subconscious and automatic activity in the body.

biofeedback, a technique aimed at changing patterns of reflex responses by behavioural conditioning based on seeing the results of previous efforts and trying to do better.

Braxton Hicks contractions, see co-ordinated contractions.

breech position, foetal position that would mean that the head was born last instead of first if untreated.

catheterisation, drawing off body fluid through a tube.

circadian rhythm, daily cycle of change in the level of some aspect of the body or its environment.

coccyx, man's vestigial tail.

co-ordinated contractions, uterine contractions that spread from cell to cell and connect up adjacent areas of the uterus.

connective tissue, fibrous body tissue that joins muscles and bones to other muscles and bones etc.

corpus luteum, ruptured egg follicle, that part of the ovary from which an egg has been released.

deoxyribonucleic acid, DNA, a string of chemical templates for making amino acids and thus different proteins including enzymes and hormones as well as muscle and bone etc.

dural tap, accidental breech into the spinal fluid contained in the spinal cord.

dystocia, literally "bad labour".

endocrine system, the hormone system, a system that manufactures and secretes substances and releases them into the blood for dispersal around the body.

endocrinology, the study of the hormone system.

endogenous, found naturally within the body.

enzyme, a biochemical catalyst for change in the structure, nature and function of biochemical substances.

epidural anaesthesia, drug delivered into the tissue around the spinal vertebrae to induce numbness.

feedback, a term borrowed from engineers describing how physical systems maintain equilibrium by measuring some aspect of the environment and taking appropriate action to maintain the status quo; for example a thermostat works using *negative* feedback, it measures room temperature and sends a message to the heater to increase heat supply if the room is too cold but sends no message if the temperature is adequate. *Positive* feedback is responsible for explosive situations, for example if a room thermostat was made to measure the temperature against some set standard and then gave instructions to turn the heat *up* instead of down if it was already hot, eventually the boiler would explode.

folic acid, a vitamin of the B complex found in leafy vegetables.

fundus, the strong muscle at the top of the uterus, see page 92

gap junctions, electrical "bridges" between cells leading to co-ordinated activity in adjacent cells.

gene, a small unit of heritable information.

genotype, an individual whose environment was absolutely perfect at supplying all the needs of a growing and living organism and provides nothing detrimental to health – an unattainable ideal organism since the environment is never perfect.

grooming, pampering oneself or someone else for the sheer pleasure of it, or for the purposes of increasing or restoring one's sense of well-being.

haemorrhage, excessive bleeding.

hypertension, high blood pressure.

hypotension, low blood pressure.

hypothalamus, the site manager of the hormone making factory, the body. Physically placed between the brain and the pituitary gland it "amplifies" signals from the brain. It can act on its own initiative but can be overruled by the brain.

hypoxia, oxygen starvation.

induction, making labour happen before body and/or mind are prepared for it.

innate, behaviour one is born with that requires no learning, for example the sucking reflex.

instinctive behaviour, behaviour that is the result of linking together innate reflex behaviours into patterns found to be a useful coping strategy.

menarche, the first menstruation.

morbidity, trauma or disease following a medical treatment or a natural event such as birth.

mortality rates, rate of death in various groups: *perinatal mortality*, babies stillborn or dying within the first week of life; *infant mortality*, babies dying before their first birthday; *maternal mortality*, mothers dying within a year of giving birth.

mutation, a change in a tiny bit of DNA leading to a change in the amino acid that bit of DNA makes, leading to a changed protein and changed cell function etc.

naloxone, a drug that reverses the effects of natural and synthetic opiates. Given to babies of mothers who have had a dose of pethidine shortly before birth.

nature/nurture controversy, how much of what we are is determined by our genes, and how much by our environnment?

neurosecretory cells, nerve cells that also secrete hormones and neurotransmitter substances.

neurotransmitters, biochemical substances involved in transmission of nervous signals.

opiates, substances that act like the drug opium. These include morphine, heroin, ß-endorphin and met-enkephalin.

paeleontology, the study of fossils.

paracrine, use of a biochemical substance near to its site of manufacture.

perineum, the area of skin and soft tissue between the vagina and the rectum.

pethidine, a narcotic opium-like drug in the same family as heroin.

phenotype, how a genotype (see above) ends up in the environnment in which he develops and lives.

Pinard stethoscope, a midwife's ear trumpet for listening to the foetal heart through the mother's abdomen.

placenta, the afterbirth, a hormone gland, the interface between maternal and foetal blood, a buffer between the mother's hormone system and the foetal hormone system.

placenta abruptio, a condition where part of the placenta has separated from the wall of the uterus.

placenta praevia, a very low-lying placenta partially or completely covering the cervix.

placental mammal, female mammals whose young are attached to them *in utero* by a umbilical cord and placenta.

pituitary gland, an amplifier of signals from the hypothalamus. The hypothalamus sends "release hormone" hormones to the pituitary and the pituitary sends instructions to hormone glands such as the ovaries and adrenal glands to increase manufacture of their own particular hormones.

For example the hypothalamus secretes CRF to the pituitary which releases ACT hormone into the blood which tells the adrenal gland to step up cortisol production.

postpartum, after birth.

prelabour, the time preceding active labour.

psychophysiology, the biology of behaviour.

psychoprophylaxis, prevention of trauma using psychological methods.

pre-eclampsia, a disorder of late pregnancy resulting in accumulation of water in body tissue, high blood pressure and protein in the urine, the new name for toxaemia. Perhaps owed to high stress hormones.

reflex, an inherited pattern of nerve firing leading to a specific physical event (for example the reflex secretion of oxytocin following stretching the vagina).

respiratory distress syndrome (RDS), a condition causing inadequate lung function owed to insufficient lung expansion and consequent lack of oxygen. Caused by lack of surfactant.

Rhesus, a blood factor first found in Rhesus monkeys, present in Rhesus positive blood and absent in Rhesus negative blood.

RU486, a drug that counteracts progesterone.

rupture of the membranes, breaking the bags containing the waters that surround the baby *in utero.*

small-for-dates, babies whose size is smaller than would be expected for the amount of time spent *in utero.*

surfactant, biochemical substance making the internal walls of the lungs less sticky.

Syntocinon, synthetic oxytocin.

Syntometrine, synthetic oxytocin with added contraction-causing chemical (ergometrine).

toxaemia, see pre-eclampsia.

Ventouse, a mechanical suction device attached to the baby's head used instead of forceps.

vertex position, where the foetus is upside down in the womb and will be born head first.

ultrasound, sonar, echogram technology, "seeing through" tissues by passing high frequency sound waves through the skin. The sound waves bounce off internal obstructions giving different patterns according to how hard the obstruction is, and thus a picture of internal conditions is built up. Ultrasound is like radar but uses sound waves instead of radio waves.

Useful Addresses

Active Birth Centre
55 Dartmouth Park Road
London NW5 1SL
071 267 3006

Association for Improvements in the Maternity Services (AIMS)
40 Kingswood Avenue, London NW6 6LS
081 960 5585

Association of Radical Midwives
62 Greetby Hill, Ormskirk
Lancashire L39 2DT
0695 72776

The British Acupuncture Association and Register
34 Alderney Street
London SW1V 4EU
071 834 1012
(Please send £2.30 for a booklet about acupuncture
and a list of practitioners).

Independent Midwives Association
94 Auckland Road
London SE19 2DB
081 771 7143

National Childbirth Trust
Alexandra House, Oldham Terrace
Acton, London W3 6NH
081 992 8637

Society to Support Home Confinements
Lydgate, Lydgate Lane
Wolsingham, Bishop Auckland
County Durham DL13 3HN
0388 528044

Women's Health Information Centre
52 Featherstone Street
London EC1Y 8RT
071 251 6580

Index